THE EGO OF INFERTILITY

COLLECTIVE

THE EGO OF INFERTILITY

STORIES OF 9 WOMEN AND
THEIR FERTILITY JOURNEY

ILLUSTRATIONS BY JACK LAFORTUNE, JIMENA DE LA VEGA

JED LAB EDITIONS INC.

JED Lab Productions inc.
Editions division

Editor: Kate Lalic
Preface by: Julie Amic
Translation and Correction: Cécile Dumortier
Artistic Director: Jack Lafortune
Illustrations: Jack Lafortune, Jimena de la Vega
Photography: Jack Lafortune

Legal Deposit, 2024 Bibliothèque et Archives Nationales du Québec

Authors :
Julie Amic
Virginie Bisson
Audrée-Anne Charron
Audrey Coutu
Geneviève Fillion
Kate Lalic
Nadine Mailloux
Sarah Milette
Virginie Paré
Sasha Plante

Title : *The Ego of Infertility: stories of 9 women and their fertility journey*
Name : *Collective*

ISBN : 978-2-9820140-3-9

Printed in Québec, Canada

To my mom, who gave me life.

TABLE OF CONTENTS

"It's not the destination, It's the journey."

—RALPH WALDO EMERSON

NINE WOMEN, NINE EGOS, NINE MONTHS

Infertility—a simple word that conceals a complex and painful reality. For many, it is a long and arduous journey, often leaving deep emotional scars. It is a story of longing and loss, of unfulfilled dreams and dashed hopes. Yet, it is also a story of courage and determination, of love and solidarity.

Infertility affects millions globally, yet it remains largely taboo and misunderstood. For many, the inability to conceive equates to shame and isolation. The silence surrounding infertility adds another layer of pain and psychological distress to an already harrowing experience.

In Canada, about one in six couples struggle to conceive. For them, access to assisted reproduction often entails obstacles, high costs, and long waiting times. Fertility treatments can be painful, stressful, and frequently do not result in the much-desired birth of a child. Despite these challenges, these couples and individuals persist in their fight to realize their dream of starting a family.

When faced with infertility, the psychological impact can be enormous. Psychological distress, depression, and anxiety are common among infertile individuals. Social and cultural pressures to start a family, along with the fear of stigma and judgment, can add an extra mental burden to an already difficult situation.

However, by breaking the silence around infertility, we can help alleviate the shame and isolation it can cause. By sharing their stories, those affected can feel less alone and find comfort within a community.

In this collective, you will discover the stories of nine courageous women who have faced the trials of infertility and assisted reproduction. Their journeys are a testament to human strength and resilience in the face of adversity. They have overcome shame and isolation and found the courage to share their experiences in their narratives. Each testimony is unique, yet they all share the rollercoaster of emotions they faced. For example, every month, they battle with hormones. They avoid baby showers at all costs and call themselves "The Hardened Ovaries Club."

Let us break the silence, the taboo, the discomfort, and the loneliness of this reality. Let us open the dialogue on infertility and assisted reproduction for men, women, and members of the LGBTQ+ community.

This book collective tells the stories of nine women going through this difficult ordeal. Each chapter offers a poignant testimony and an example of resilience. Each of these women has faced challenging choices, moments of discouragement and despair. They have known sadness, anger, frustration, and disappointment. But they have also known love, joy, and hope. This book is an open-hearted testimony. We followed the unfiltered daily lives of nine fighters determined to overcome adversity to achieve their dream of motherhood. It is a story of hope and life, a story that deserves to be told.

To these nine exceptional fighters, who had the courage to share their personal stories with all of us, I am deeply grateful. Their strength, resilience, and determination have illuminated my path and inspire each of us to face adversity with courage and grace.

My love, Koko, your loving and comforting presence gave me the strength to keep moving forward, even when I was overwhelmed by the tumultuous waves of uncertainty.

To Annabel and Alex, my beacons in the darkness, your wisdom and kindness gave me the hope to continue, even when everything seemed lost.

PREFACE

By Julie Amic, Doula

To those of you who sit with heavy hearts as you read this book, perhaps seeking a glimmer of hope or emotional validation, or simply curious to know if others share similar experiences, I offer my heartfelt understanding. Regardless of your reason, I am convinced that you will find what you came looking for. They are nine, but you are thousands. Each with your own challenges, stories, reactions, emotions... However, one thing unites you all: fragmentation. It's the profound tearing that leads to a detachment from the real world, a sensation of leaving your body only to return, reborn. For each of you, there was a moment, a precise instant when you realized that your journey would be different. Everything turned monochrome, shattered, and in that brokenness, you found the strength to rebuild and move forward on your uncertain path to motherhood.

Until recently, I was a woman like many people in your circle, meaning someone who was uninformed about the issues of infertility. I personally had the privilege of easily conceiving my children. My idea of "what if I couldn't" conceive so easily was limited to the sadness that this thought provoked in me. In my youth and young adulthood, no one ever told me that it was a possibility, that infertility was a real issue for many women. I knew it existed, but I had no idea what it all entailed.

I will always remember the day my world awakened to your reality. It was during a baby shower. My surprise pregnancy was guessed and awkwardly revealed by a woman from our group of friends.

She said loudly, "OMG JULIE! You don't want any wine? You must be pregnant!"

Those who know me, know how bad of a liar I am. The discomfort and surprise caught me off guard, and I simply responded with a discreet "yes." Instantly, I experienced a discomfort I did not quite grasp. I froze; I was happy but embarrassed.

One of my friends present that day, already a natural mother, had been trying to conceive again for almost two years without success. She and her partner had even started a process to try to find a reason for this new infertility situation. That day, I opened myself a little more to her reality and understood all the nuances of the emotions she was feeling. In her eyes, without a word being spoken, I saw the complexity of her happiness for me, but also her jealousy, anger, sorrow, guilt, and everything that comes with it. A few days later, we talked about how the situation made us feel. She felt guilty for not being able to fully rejoice in my happiness; she had to face her wounds. I felt bad for having this unfair ease in getting pregnant and couldn't fully experience my happiness for fear of hurting her more. Out of love for each other, we chose to take a break from our friendship. I was sad, but I understood that she needed this space. Today, her second daughter is about to turn two, and we are closer than ever. My children call her "Auntie." She is a happy woman and a fulfilled mother who has made peace with this period of her life, which has made her stronger and more resilient than ever.

After my maternity leave, I worked in a private clinic as a nursing assistant for pregnant women. I met women every day who shared their stories with me. Without knowing it, all these exchanges and discussions would influence my professional journey. It was as if a veil had been lifted, and I realized how much more numerous you are than we are led to believe. I realized that my friend's story is common. I was shocked by the lack of awareness. That's how my own awareness began. Subsequently, I quickly felt a strong urge to resume my private doula practice to offer a little gentleness to women with an atypical journey to motherhood. And, naturally, without seeking, they came to me.

Virginie. Kate. Maude. Natasha. Marie. Isabelle. Noemie.

For all these women that life will put on your path, thank you for taking the time to read this collection and raising awareness. The resistance you will feel as you go through their stories is part of the process. Continue nonetheless. The awareness that your reading will bring will dissipate your discomfort and leave room for a much more empathetic and compassionate stance. And to you, dear mother in the making, I wish you to find what you came looking for, whatever your reason. Whether it's to find the strength to continue to believe in your motherhood project or to fully experience your fragmentation in order to rise stronger. I wish you to find the resilience to accept that your story is valid and that it can be beautiful, even if it's different.

Give yourself the right to doubt, to be afraid, and to feel helpless at times. Give yourself also the right to laugh and to fully experience the joys of everyday life, because that's exactly what motherhood is; the greatest paradox of a lifetime.

CHAPTER 1

MAKING A BABY, NOT SO EASY

By Kate Lalic

As I settle in at the chalet, coffee in hand, a glimmer of excitement brightens my eyes. An enlightenment, just like in fairy tales. Why not share our stories? For our well-being and as an inspiration to other women who are going through this journey with us. Strangely, this secret, I keep it to myself. For three years, I've been on a fertility journey, and my Instagram feed remains undisturbed. I openly share my travels, my private life, my entrepreneurial ventures, but never have I been able to open up about this life challenge that's been thrown my way. It's caused me to retreat, and I kept this secret until last year. The day I confessed to my parents that I already had three embryos in storage, their faces fell. They were astonished that I hadn't said anything, that I had kept it all to myself, and experienced the most poignant emotions of my life without their support. Their first question was, "Why didn't you say anything?

— "Shame," I believe I whispered, between tears.

The burden of the grief I carried; too heavy to simply be tucked away. Bent under this weight, I carry sorrow, shame, injustice and a feeling of dishonor, all trapped in this agonizingly slow race against time. 30 years old, no children of my own.

Over the past three years, I've lost friends, I've lied, I've hidden, and I've portrayed a false reality of my life on social media. This secret was mine, and I'm not one to reveal everything. However, with hindsight, I see how communication and sharing my fertility journey could help someone else bear their burden. The purpose of this book: to gather testimonies, stories, and experiences of infertility from nine unique women who share the same desire, to bring life into the world. Whatever form the miracle may take, we desire to become mothers...

After my second decaffeinated coffee, I reach out to Julie, the doula. She believes in the project and starts gathering women who would like to open up and explore the possibility of supporting others in their own fertility journey. I jump on the phone and write to Alexandra, my anchor in this adventure:

"Alex, there is a fine line between genius and insanity, but this time around, I believe this project can truly have a major impact. The anonymous texts I've written on your blog, let's publish them openly. Let's gather women, their stories, and lift the veil. I'm ready."

My heart bursts with happiness when I see her response appear a few minutes later: "GO. Let's do this."

With utmost tenderness, I started this project that will lead to the publication of this book. Blogging anonymously about my fertility journey gave me the courage to bare myself. I appreciated the response from other women, their comments, and their support. I felt compelled to create a collection that brings together the stories of women like me, with different paths. We're all on this adventure, with our own battles. Without vulnerability, there is no courage. To you reading these lines, never forget that your vulnerability is a strength. Have courage through this storm, we support you, lift you up. The road is shorter together, you are not alone. What I've learned from the fertility journey is difficult to apply, but at the same time so simple: You have to embrace this experience, as the journey is magical with its ups and downs.

SEPTEMBER 2021

I spread out the syringes, vials, bandages, disinfectant, and instructions on the bed. I, who hadn't taken advanced science classes in fifth grade, am now doing so at an accelerated pace. My hands tremble at this grand spectacle of medication and injections. I take my cell phone out of my pocket to capture this moment. This photo, which will not leave my phone, represents the beginning of an adventure.

"Are you ready?" Koko says, poking his head through the doorway.

"Yes, one more minute. I'm going to transfer the powder into the liquid and prepare the syringe."

I take a deep breath and open the plastic wrap; it's a start! I hear the phone ringing in the distance. I can hear a familiar voice on the other end; it's his brother calling.

"Yeah, everything alright? We're at the cottage for the weekend."

I strain to listen. Unfortunately, we had to miss a family party today, and with the start of the injections, we had to make ourselves scarce.

"How was the party?" Koko continues.

I hear him going down the stairs. As I can no longer hear the rest of the conversation, I focus on my task. Okay, after transferring the liquid into the powder, what's the next step?

His footsteps echo in the hallway.

"It was my brother."

"Oh yeah?" I say innocently. "Was the party good?"

"They're going to have a second child. Lola is pregnant."

My body stiffens. I feel like crap. How can I not have a lump in my throat? Happy for the expanding family, the beautiful moments, and the welcome of this new child, but stunned that it's hitting us today. What were the odds of starting an IVF cycle and receiving this news from his brother at the same time?

He sits on the edge of the bed and turns to me. His face is stoic. I can't read anything through his coal-black eyes. No emotion emanates from him, just like a doctor lifting a scalpel.

"Are you ready?"

"Yes," I say with the voice of a five-year-old who's just been told to stop crying.

I don't even dare to respond or discuss the news. Maybe we'll never talk about it again. For now.

He takes the syringe from my hands, removes the cap delicately, and approaches my belly. I quickly close my eyes to avoid seeing the needle pierce my flesh. I pinch my stomach with my hands to guide it to the right spot: not too close to the belly button, but not too far either!

The needle pierces my skin and the pain sets in. I can feel the liquid slowly descending, a warmth spreading through my body like lightning, flames entering my veins. My eyelashes hold back my tears; I can't hold back the tears any longer. The pressure and the pain are unbearable.

"It's almost done... actually, it's done!"

He removes the needle and, hands shaking, he tries to secure it with the cap. Unfortunately, he misses the needle, pricking the tip of his finger.

"Ouch! Damn it, I just pricked my finger with the syringe!" he says, startled.

His tone changes and panic sets in.

"My finger is starting to heat up, this isn't normal. It needs to be disinfected right away. It's swelling!"

I rush to the bathroom, holding my belly with one hand to apply a Paw Patrol bandage (yes, I bought children's Band-Aids to lighten the mood).

"Let me apply some alcohol."

I sit by his side, holding his hands. He seems completely bewildered. It's certainly the call from his brother that makes our first experience memorable.

The scene could have been written for the movies. Two lovers on the edge of the bed, amidst syringes, alcohol swabs, and medications in an atmosphere that breathes despair. On the verge of tears, they embraced to forget this scene. Cut!

My fertility journey began a year before the pandemic. It had been five years since I stopped using contraception. Were we careful? Yes and no! We got engaged, then married, both on cloud nine, we knew we wanted to start a family. Just before the first wave of COVID-19 hit Quebec, we had THE conversation.

"OK, so are we really trying?"

"Yes... I can't wait to have a baby with you, my wife. We're ready."

Those words stayed with me for a few days, imprinted in the palm of my hand. My heart was bursting with joy; I would soon be a mother. A title I had desired since I was a little girl. I had always told myself that my life would truly begin when I had a family. For now, my family is you, Koko. You and me, facing the storm ahead.

My first laparoscopy and right fallopian tube ablation took place on July 15, 2021.

I remember a pandemic evening, when everyone was glued to Netflix, TikTok, and live podcasts on social media. My husband, involved in several projects as a director, was collaborating on a podcast that presented topics related to sexuality. One of the hosts was talking about not wanting children. My husband, very proud of the baby project we had started, that is, "trying for real," mentioned it on the air. The two hosts looked at each other, and a moment of heavy silence ensued.

"Oh, that's fine. But, if I were you, I might not say it. You know, just in case it doesn't work out or takes longer. Keep your secret."

And I believe it was at that moment, when I heard that conversation through the door, that a knot formed in my stomach. The ego of infertility. What if it didn't work out?

A few days earlier, I had missed a FaceTime call from a childhood friend, Emma. I was in line at Starbucks. I had a feeling she wanted to tell me something. It's not like her to Facetime. Did she want to see a reaction? Discuss a problem? A lightning bolt flashed before my eyes. Oh! She's pregnant, I thought. She wants to share the good news with me. I was waiting for my iced coffee and tapping on my phone with one hand.

"You're pregnant? Oh, wow."

"How did you know? I'll call you back."

My face fell. I was speechless.

"Kate, iced coffee, two pumps of vanilla."

I grabbed the glass, my fingers numb. Was it the ice or the overflowing emotions that made my fingertips tingle? Making my way to the terrace, I called her back.

"How did you know?" she exclaimed.

Her face was radiant and her excitement palpable.

"I don't know, I just had a feeling," I told her, absorbing the good news. "But I didn't know you were trying. You must be so happy!"

"That's the craziest part, we're not trying at all. In fact, I had an IUD, and it happened, just like that! We didn't expect it at all."

She seemed nervous, maybe scared by this adventure that was beginning.

"I'm so happy for you, you know, we're trying too! I think we could be pregnant at the same time; it would be amazing. We could go for walks, yoga classes, etc."

I was already projecting into the future to reassure her (and myself) that we could make it together.

Summer was drawing to a close, and my periods continued to arrive like clockwork. My morale was decreasing along with the cooling autumn air.

MY FIRST INSEMINATION TOOK PLACE IN SEPTEMBER 2021.

It failed. I dreaded starting the injections process again. I was more apprehensive about taking medications than the insemination itself.

Taking hormones is the worst step, in my opinion. It's also the longest. Hormones orally, hormones vaginally, hormones in injections... all of which in the course of two weeks.

Then comes the big day, followed by two more weeks of waiting. And then, we start over!

I felt tired, depressed, anxious... In the past, I had struggled with anxiety. Negative thoughts resurfaced, and I felt out of control. Even yoga couldn't ease my mind anymore. The day of the insemination carries with it a profound significance and an undeniable strangeness. Your mind tells you, "This is it!" and your body tells you, "This isn't natural..."

Lying on the table, I endure the recommended twenty minutes after the procedure. Koko scrolls down YouTube videos to fill the time, while I am in shock from the emotion. Or lack thereof. It's done so mechanically. It's all in the hands of science. At this moment, I realized my journey was neither easy nor magical. I held back my tears because my heart refused to accept that our journey to conception wasn't on Egyptian cotton sheets, but rather on wax paper.

AFTER MY SECOND INSEMINATION, NOVEMBER 2021

My period started on the day I was supposed to take the pregnancy test. As if I didn't believe it, I still took the test. Koko and I were on a business trip to Toronto; we had to keep our heads held high. As if not to feel anything, I put my tears aside and my emotions in a small imaginary drawer, for later. I'm not sure it was a good thing.

I had so many questions: Is this the right time? Would I be a good mom? Should I continue with the procedures? I thought about this "potential motherhood" at least once a day, with moments of uncertainty and sadness. Nevertheless, I tried to push these thoughts out of my mind.

I was told that the more you thought about it, the more stressed you became, and the lower the chances were.

I didn't talk about it. I was afraid people would pity me or judge me. Not to mention the infamous question that would come up every month: "So, are you pregnant?" If my relatives had known, it would have added stress on me. On the other hand, I found myself naturally withdrawing from acquaintances who had just given birth or become pregnant... those who had strong opinions on the subject as well. Since it tended to undermine my spirits and give me even more reasons to compare myself, I distanced myself. Probably not to suffer. It's instinctive. Keeping the secret. When I saw pregnancy announcements, gender reveal parties, and received calls from a cousin and a sister-in-law to announce their good news on social media, I swallowed my tears. Congratulating them, I confronted my feelings of injustice. Visits to the clinic for the protocol led me to accumulate white lies. Justifying absences, avoiding alcohol-filed events, pretending...

I feel a bit like Carrie Bradshaw in the episode of Sex and the City where she decides to create a gift registry for her shoes given the number of baby showers and children's parties she has to attend. Why not celebrate as well? Am I going to remain the "cool aunt" for life?

I gently knock on Annie's door.

"Come in, my dear," she says through the door.

I enter silently because I don't know what to say after a weekend of pretending to enjoy life.

"Tell me, how were your past two weeks?"

I look into her deep blue eyes and exhale. Inhale. Exhale. How lucky I am to have this woman in my life, my therapist.

She keeps me grounded and safe minded. Her calm energy dissipates my anxiety in an instant.

"The insemination didn't work," I say.

She looks at me intensely to soothe my sorrow. Inhale. Exhale.

"Everyone around me is pregnant. It happened all of a sudden. Koko and I are trying to navigate this new fertility universe. I don't know what awaits us, especially since we're keeping it a secret."

"You don't feel comfortable talking about it?"

"Not yet, it's too painful. It's like I'm going through the stages of grief: shock, denial, anger, depression, resignation, acceptance, and rebuilding. I might be in the denial stage right now."

"Yes, I understand. Do you think you can reach the acceptance stage?"

"I believe so, especially with my new project. I had the idea to gather nine women who are going through fertility struggles. Each of them would write a chapter to share their story. Like a therapy circle, we'd meet every month to work on the project. Through their stories, I soften my pain. They help me move forward."

"It's your support network, Kate; keep going in this direction."

I smile and watch her take notes. Maybe this anthology will help thousands of women? And perhaps by the time it's completed, I'll have my own miracle in my belly?

MARCH 2021

The cold, waxed table gave me chills.

"I see a mass, but don't worry."

"The words "mass" and "worry" in the same sentence don't bode well." Suddenly, I felt very hot. I stammered timidly, "Is it cancer?"

"No, I don't believe so, but we'll need to proceed with an exploratory surgery", was I answered bluntly.

A few months later and one fallopian tube less...

JULY 2021

Naked in front of the mirror, I observed my scars. These four incisions on my stomach reminded me of the moment when I had to make the decision to go under the procedure. I wished I could hide in a wardrobe and hold my breath so no one would find me. The evil eye of infertility pulled me out of hiding and brought me back to reality.

When I stood at the altar and vowed to be present in sickness and in health, I never thought fate would make me comply so quickly. I will always look after my husband... but the problem, in this instance, was me, my own body. It couldn't give life without the help of science. Every day was a battle in my mind, and ego always triumphed over reason.

"How do you feel?" A question that comes up often these days. When I tried to explain to Koko the feelings that haunted me, I found myself at a loss. I lacked the words to convey the storm that raged within me. Drowning in a sea of guilt, I struggled to breathe as tears flowed. Why me? This question looped in my head. One less fallopian tube, four scars, and a wounded heart. I couldn't shake the guilt that weighed heavily on me, especially in the presence of my husband. Knowing he could start a family with someone else naturally, without having to go through this obstacle, I couldn't help but blame my body and constantly scrutinize my reflection in the mirror. Guilt consumed me. Yet, he remained a constant source of reassurance.

"Don't worry, you'll be a mother one day," he repeated, always kind-hearted.

Not worrying... A sport I had been practicing since this summer. A bicycle racing full speed in my mind, one I couldn't control. The ego of infertility was catching up to me; it was right behind me! Hormones blurred my vision, and the injections were so strong they numbed me. Hiding under the covers, I muffled the sound of my distress. I didn't want him to know. He already saw too much. Too many tears, too much anxiety, too many setbacks.

"Madam, if you want a chance to conceive, we must start a protocol quickly." A striking phrase. I searched for a hint of empathy in the tone of the voice, to no avail. I see myself, as a child, feeding my little sister. I see myself, at eighteen, telling my parents that my dream is to be a stay-at-home mom. I see myself, at twenty-eight, crossing my fingers every month. Then, I look at myself today, at thirty, facing the mirror, confronting the greatest fear of my life. A nightmare turned into reality, one that I can't control. And my ego was incapable of digesting it.

APRIL 2022

This morning, I had a panic attack. The kind of moment when everything collapses. Words fail to explain the internal tearing and the sadness that rose in me like the tide of the Atlantic. It rushes in and pulls me into the darkest depths.

That day, I decided to play on two fronts and give it my all. I will be on two waiting lists simultaneously. Like the saying goes, I could kill two birds with one stone. I sent an application to a new clinic.

Their email response mentioned a three-month wait. Okay. It had been 4 months on the other, never ending waiting list and it was making me sick.

The good news in all of this: I had stopped taking hormones since December. The effects had dissipated, and I was starting to regain control of my body. However, my mind was still filled with negative thoughts.

I panicked and called Annie to schedule an appointment. She had a cancellation. Koko drove me to her office. My hands were shaking, and my vision was blurred. I didn't know who to turn to nor where to go. I had lost my way. Nobody was steering the ship, and the tide was catching up to me. I had never cried in front of her, nor in front of my friends. Not even in front of my mother. The storm was inside me. I sat down in front of her and began:

"Did you know that the first test-tube baby in Quebec was my neighbor?"

She crossed her legs, leaned back in her chair, and said, "Tell me."

Her slight smile let me know that she saw through my stories. She saw my strength, my resilience, and, above all, a sense of humor that I definitely hadn't lost.

"I was five years old. I remember it so vividly. I was riding my pink bicycle when I lost control and fell to the ground. My knee was bleeding, and I panicked and cried until he appeared, like a knight in shining armor. He saw me on the sidewalk and came to rescue me. He was tall, with brown hair. He scooped me up, carrying me home like a princess. It was quite literally my first crush!"

"In your opinion, what is the moral of this story?"

"That if you fall, you should always get back up, and that you can also rely on the people around you for help... Don't be afraid to ask."

— Exactly, she said with a wink.

My heart felt lighter. Despite the setbacks and their inevitable scars, I must continue to move forward. I don't know what became of my knight, the IVF baby. Life works in mysterious ways.

MAY 2022

Mother's Day. For the first time, this day was excruciatingly painful. Our agenda was filled with a family brunch and a visit from a newborn. I begged Koko to let me stay home. Reluctantly, feeling like a zombie, I spent the day with a fake smile and a heavy heart. The emotional effort to leave my cocoon was tremendous. No one suspected anything. It was as if Koko and I were putting on a show, scene after scene. I repeated the same lines, the same emotions, so as not to break character. I hoped not to go through this again next year.

JULY 2022

One year after my initial surgery and two failed inseminations later, the anticipation for the clinics to reopen, after COVID 19's sanitary restrictions, becomes agonizing. I finally received a phone call. Was it a sign? I want to believe it was. I'll take any semblance of hope as a sign of fate. I avoided walking under a ladder and feared black cats. Superstition takes over when hope is lost.

"Madam, your first appointment will be on August 19th."

"Really?"

The words lingered in the air.

"Make sure not to forget your medical file."

Said file was right in front of me, on my desk. 189 pages of ultrasounds, results, blood tests, protocols, semen analysis, disappointments, and sufferings. I push the file aside and focus on my work. My phone rings again. It's Emma. I don't have the strength to answer her and listen to her joys and sorrows as a new mother. Unfortunately, through this ordeal, I lost a friend. I haven't told her that her sweet moments of motherhood cause me anxiety. I try to avoid her. I know that one day our paths will cross again and I will be able to explain everything to her. For now, I have no words. Emma, I'm sorry.

AUGUST 2022

— I see that your file is complete. You can start the IVF protocol in your next cycle. There's no more waiting, Madam," she said, turning towards me.

She could see my glassy eyes filled with tears, a sight she most likely encountered daily. Behind my mask, my lower lip trembled. I clutched my purse tightly, my hands shaking. What was I experiencing? A fresh start, perhaps. Emotions were swirling within me. First, the potential joy of having a baby in my belly, but then the sadness, even mourning, of not conceiving a little one naturally. The excitement of the steps to come and the days ticking away on the calendar. And the fear. Always that fear. The fear of disappointment, the fear of injections twice a day, the fear of being unable to carry life. My head was spinning, but my heart was still beating a little louder this morning.

SEPTEMBER 2022

With a smile on my face, the worst was almost behind me. I had one more week of injections left, and then the famous egg retrieval.

An intervention during which they suction all the eggs ready to be fertilized in the laboratory. We arrived at the clinic for one final ultrasound before the retrieval. My eggs must have been quite ready, because my belly felt like it was going to burst. I was so swollen, I even had bruises on my stomach, and my breasts overflowed from my bra. There are good and bad sides to it. It's a little taste of pregnancy, they say!

"Kate, room 2 for the ultrasound."

The nurse was familiar, given the number of times we had spoken on the phone and exchanged emails. I thought I might suggest brunch next time! I talked to her more often than to my friends. Hand in hand with Koko, we made our way to the room. I sat down on the wax paper, full of hope. The doctor had a strange look on his face. His expression changed as he rolled the cold tool back and forth, to make sure of what he was seeing... a mass.

"I'm sorry, we won't be able to proceed with the embryo transfer after your retrieval. We'll have to freeze the embryos and plan for surgery."

"But..."

I couldn't speak; the tears were already welling up. I dared not turn to Koko; he squeezed my hand. I knew he felt my pain at that very moment. He didn't want to see me go through surgery again. The doctor continued the explanation, too logical for my feelings:

"We need to remove the left tube and ensure that everything is ready to receive an embryo. Your left tube is swollen with harmful fluid, and we need to confirm the presence of a mass. Surgery will be the best solution at this stage. We don't want to compromise the embryos. Continue the injections, and we'll proceed with the retrieval. We'll freeze the embryos and wait for your body to heal."

I fell apart. Another surgery... Both fallopian tubes no longer attached to my body. How could two small tubes affect me so much? I only had one left, and it had just let me down.

"I'll send the request today. We hope everything will go quickly. Everything will be fine, it's not a serious case. One month after the operation, we'll proceed with the implantation. Don't worry."

The thread of hope I clung to was severed with a sharp blow. I sensed a shift in my husband, a subtle weakening of his once-unwavering strength, as if the armor of his resilience was slowly chipping away. It pierced me to the core. Since we started our fertility journey, our love has evolved, unbreakable. Yet, the next months would be harder, darker. For me, the retrieval marked the final step towards the end of this process. But it turns out to be the beginning of another process and a waiting period in the healthcare system.

"We'll make it, I'm here with you," he whispered, looking at me with intensity.

He truly believed it, and I had no choice but to believe it as well.

RETRIEVAL DAY

The injections were finally over! Three injections a day to reach this great day: the egg retrieval. I'll spare you the details, but it was a challenging step. I wear the wool socks my grandmother had given me as a gift. She always told me to keep my feet warm and insisted on putting socks on me every time I came back home. These socks are my lucky charm today. I'm sure she's watching over me.

It was freezing cold in the OR. Everything was blurry; I could hear voices in the distance and instruments clanging on metal. My husband was close to me; he ran his hand through my hair and told me everything was okay. I heard little, but I felt everything. Without moving, I endured the pain. Suddenly, I felt warmth in my right arm: another dose to calm me down.

I don't remember much aside from the number: eleven.

Eleven eggs were retrieved. The embryologist, who was on the other side of a window in the operating room, exclaimed:

"We have eleven, congratulations!"

Eleven is a good number, I thought to myself, closing my eyes and praying. I fell asleep peacefully, under the effects of the sedation.

DAY 2

The embryologist called and confirmed eight fertilized eggs... So, eight embryos were developing. Wow! A whole football team! Our smiles gradually returned...

DAY 4

We had five still developing. We lost the others along the way. Nature follows its process. With crossed fingers, I waited for the embryologist's last call on day 5...

DAY 5

"You have three perfect embryos ready to be frozen!" she said on the phone. "They're of excellent quality on the chart, and all three are ready for implantation."

Our looks said it all; we hugged and held on for a long moment. Our hearts were filled with happiness. See you soon, my three darlings.

OCTOBER 2022

Upon landing, we retrieved our luggage, and headed home, feeling feverish. After two weeks under the sun of the Côte d'Azur, the return to reality hit hard. The next morning, I had to go to the hospital for an MRI. Koko accompanied me; I didn't think I could go alone. I was terrified of this metallic monster that swallows you whole in its mouth. My stomach clenches just thinking about it. I've always loved roller coasters, extreme rides, but the MRI machine gives me shivers. It reminds me of my grandmother's cancer, my great-grandmother's, and more recently, my mother's. She had a mass on her ovary that was detected and quickly removed. I'm next, I tell myself. I don't say anything to Koko, and I keep my worries to myself. Especially after such a magical trip.

Besides infertility, which has defined me for the past two years, my life is full of projects, beauty, and opportunities. We live a double life. Behind this facade of exciting projects and jet-set life hides hormone injections in the bathroom at social events, tears, and lots of raspberry leaf tea. Uncertainty gnaws at us, but we keep hope alive...

Still jet lagged, we arrived at the hospital, where I was asked to change into a "pretty" blue gown. Can we get some designers on this project? I'd love to see this garment revamped! It is so drab and uncomfortable. I wasn't in the best of moods in the small dressing room. They called my number coldly over the microphone.

"Number 752."

I quickly tied the gown, grabbed my boots, and put on the hair cap. Quite a look! Koko watched me walk down the hallway with a ghostly expression.

"We need to go here, Madam," they said, pointing to a chair with blood draw equipment next to it.

"Why? Is there another test to do?" I asked suspiciously.

"Yes, we need to administer some intravenous fluids before the MRI."

I burst into tears. Unable to hold back, I exploded. My nose was running, my cheeks were flushed, my breath was short.

"You can't have an anxiety attack now, Kate, you'll be entering the machine soon, and you can't move at all," Koko said nervously.

"I can't take it anymore. I might have cancer," I blurted out. I was filled with rage. I couldn't bear any more tests, needles, decisions made for me, being told what to do every week for two years. I couldn't take it anymore. I wanted to scream, to thrash, to lie down in the gray hallway. Listen to me, I can't take it anymore...

NOVEMBER 2022

The day of the second surgery, the laparoscopic salpingectomy, the removal of my left fallopian tube and the extraction of a six-centimeter mass.

The cold glow of the neon lights twinkled in the hospital room, painting the walls a pale and gloomy hue. Lying on the bed, my fingers cautiously touched the bandage covering my abdomen, as if I could feel the pain through this thick layer of cotton. Kate... The name echoed in my head like a distant echo, as if the person I was before this operation was nothing but a faded memory.

Today, I lost much more than my last fallopian tube. I lost a part of myself, a part of my identity as a woman. The announcement of the six-centimeter mass growing inside me was a blow, shattering the dreams of motherhood I had cherished for so long. Every heartbeat now seems suffocated by a sense of sadness and despair. At thirty-two years old, an age when one should feel accomplished, satisfied with their achievements. And yet, here, in this sterile room, I felt torn apart by a bitter sense of failure. The laparoscopic salpingectomy... A medical term that sounded like an unforgiving sentence. The left and right of my feminine being were now incomplete, deprived of their fallopian tubes. How had I come to this point? My life had seemed beautiful, filled with projects and successes, but I found myself facing a bitter paradox. Luck had seemed to smile upon me, granting me so much, but that same luck seemed to deny me the very essence of femininity I had always desired: to become a mother.

The scars left by this ordeal multiplied, both on my body and in my heart. My belly now bore the visible marks of this surgical intervention, but it was the invisible scars that hurt the most. These emotional wounds that made me doubt my future fertility, that filled me with fears and uncertainties. I closed my eyes, trying to banish the dark thoughts that assailed me and the post-operative nausea. Koko was by my side. His comforting words tried to heal my inner wounds, but he could not grasp the full extent of my pain. To him, the scars on my belly were minimal, but to me, they were gigantic.

As the silence of the recovery room enveloped me, a flow of tears streamed down my cheeks. I felt lost, like a soul searching for meaning in all of this. The shadows of my femininity seemed to suffocate me, and in that darkness, I desperately searched for a glimmer of hope, a way to reinvent my path despite this heart-wrenching ordeal. We both share the same pain. A pain I had seen in Koko's eyes, moments before the nurse wheeled me to the operating room. As I turned my head to catch a glimpse of him before surgery, I saw the anguish etched in his deep, black eyes. Helpless in that moment, the image of his sorrow is one I will never forget.

THE FALLOPIAN MONOLOGUE

I listened to Charlotte Cardin's song "Phoenix" on repeat and tried to write, hoping to ease my pain. One dose at a time, I'm taking the prescribed blue narcotics. Not too much, but not enough to forget the pain. Outside, the first snowflakes were falling. They were heavy and fell slowly, much like I felt at the moment... My swollen, bloated belly was unforgiving. I pushed my laptop onto my lap to avoid discomfort. I thought of Émile Nelligan and his garden of frost. He influences my writing, and between his moments of lucidity and delirium, I can see the beauty of winter. The garden of frost surrounded me; it's the right time to rest. Two weeks ahead of me to slow down and to take time; time to breathe and heal my wounds, my soul... Although stormy thoughts sneak in between my naps, I inhale and exhale.

It has been seven days since I lost the choice. The choice to conceive life 100% naturally. Medically, there was no choice. Mentally, it was paralysis. Drained, I was tired, and my heart knotted. I discovered and untangled feminist movements, women's suffrage, gender equality. Nature had robbed me. Reluctantly, I accepted it slowly, as slowly as the snowflakes falling around my frosty garden. I witnessed my white orchid wanting to bloom again, to be born a second time. I closely observed the three buds. Was it a sign? I want to see the signs when they appear. They were before my eyes, my three babies. Our three buds will bloom...

Koko saw me, eyes filled with water, looking out the window with a barely touched cup of tea. He approached and cuddled me, his head on my shoulder. He needed comfort as well. He tries to reassure me, to convince me that my scars are insignificant in his eyes, that I am beautiful, that nothing has changed for him. Yet, despite all his good intentions, he cannot understand the psychological pain that accompanies the loss of my two fallopian tubes.

Koko, my love, I wish you could understand the magnitude of this loss. It's as if you lost both your testicles, imagine for a moment that reality. A brutal vision, I know. But that's equivalent to what I'm going through. It's as if I'm being deprived of the very essence of my femininity.

The days passed by slowly since the operation. Finally, the time had come to remove the bandages that protected my scars. A part of me wanted to see, wanted to face reality, while another part trembled at the thought of discovering these marks that had forever changed the landscape of my body. With a hesitant hand, I removed the first bandage, revealing the first scar. My breath caught in my throat, as if I had witnessed a surgery without consent. It was there, minimal, but already different from the first operation. The second time was always harder, deeper, as if the body remembered, as if the soul carried the burden of the past.

Tears blurred my vision as I undid the remaining bandages, revealing the other scars stretching across my belly. They echoed each other, like sisters wounded by the same fate. The fine lines, witnesses of modern medicine, seemed to contradict the magnitude of the turmoil they represented for me.

These scars, both physical and mental, were now a part of me. They told a story of struggle, resilience, but also vulnerability. I wished to see them fade, to vanish with time, but instead, they seemed to anchor themselves further, forcing me to confront a reality I had not chosen. It was the second time I had to face this sight, the second time I found myself facing my reflection, fragmented, raw from life. The tears continued to flow, silent witnesses of my pain and strength at the same time. Because despite everything, these scars had not erased my will to rise, to seek meaning in this ordeal, to find new ways to express my femininity.

So, with a glimmer of determination in my eyes, I embrace these scars as evidence of my resilience, of my ability to overcome adversity. I was not broken, but shaped by the trials that had forged the woman I became. And if the scars were to be exposed in broad daylight, I would know how to wear them with grace, for they are now part of my story, of my journey towards an unexpected rebirth.

The vibration of my phone snapped me out of my trance. I received a message from my brother as he was on his way to come help me at the cottage after my surgery. My head was still confused and dizzy.

"Do you want some chocolate?" he asked.

Just the thought of it filled me with joy, so I gladly accepted his offer.

My brother understands post-operative pain, as he has also undergone a similar operation: a total laparoscopic hysterectomy. He chose to take control of his body, his transition, and his struggles related to gender dysphoria. By reducing the long-term risks of cancer, the surgery was also the best decision for his physical and psychological health. Niko was once my sister, but he bravely decided to follow his heart and become the man he was always meant to be. I am proud of him for having the courage to live his truth, despite the challenges he had to face. His transition was a struggle to find his identity, a battle to align his body with his mind, but he overcame it with strength and determination. Now, he is finally free to live his authentic life, in charge of his destiny. This operation meant liberation and control over his body and his anxiety related to gender dysphoria. Fertility stories also affect men, transgender individuals, and the LGBTQ2S+ community.[1]

---

1 The issue of fertility is often considered a domain reserved for women, but this couldn't be further from the truth. Men, transgender individuals, and the LGBTQ2S+ community are also affected by this complex and emotional issue. For many of us, fertility is intimately linked to our gender identity and our relationship with our bodies. For transgender individuals, fertility choices can be particularly challenging, as they may involve giving up their ability to conceive or undergoing expensive and invasive treatments to preserve this ability. But whatever decision we make, the issue of fertility is an important aspect of our lives that deserves to be treated with respect and understanding.

DECEMBER 2022

December arrived quietly with its first blanket of snow. I anxiously awaited for the biopsy results, fearing the worst and hoping for the best. Sitting at a café, I was about to meet with a producer from California about some writing projects. A meeting that was meant to be positive after the difficult convalescence. It was my first outing in town and in jeans! Yes! I finally managed to put on jeans since my belly was much less swollen. My phone vibrated on the wooden table; it was an unknown number. I answered quickly.

"Yes?"

"It's the nurse from the hospital, calling to give you the results of the mass biopsy. It was a large 6-centimeter mass."

I dared not to breathe. She continued.

"And it's benign."

"Really? Okay, what wonderful news, just before Christmas! Thank you, thank you for this call," I said with excitement.

"I wish you a speedy recovery and a happy holiday season with peace of mind!"

I breathed out heavily. Phew. I dodged a bullet. I'm okay, I'm okay. I can stop the anxiety. I felt relieved, and finally, I smiled for the first time in months.

JANUARY 2023

As I wrote these lines, I believed I was pregnant. I had been carrying life for five days, and I was so proud. On the day of the embryo transfer, I arrived at the clinic in my best outfit, my lucky warm socks (which my grandmother gave me just before her passing), and a beautiful energy. I believed in it. We saw it on the screen, under the microscope. He (or she) was perfectly round, beautiful, and perfect. A 3AA embryo, which means, in fertility jargon, an excellent embryo.

We were full of hope as we watched the embryo slide into the cavity of my uterus. Whispering to my husband, I asked, "Do you think you could film the moment to keep a memory and show it to him when he grows up?"

A miracle of science. We held hands, held our breath, and then it was done.

"Okay, it's done!" the doctor said enthusiastically. You could hear the satisfaction in his voice. Confidence radiated from him.

"Come back to see me in 18 months, because I just dropped off a boy for you, and you can come back for your girl."

We all laughed a bit to lighten the mood; even the nurse was smiling behind her mask. It certainly wasn't the first time she had heard that joke! I relaxed for a while, then thought about the two-week wait before the blood test. What would I do to pass the time? I made myself a schedule: morning meditation, cut off social media, read in bed at night, line up outings and business meetings, do a special grocery shopping for the ingredients mentioned in my thousands of Google searches, get acupuncture, etc. My mind raced quickly, like when you pick up speed in a bike race. It's scary, but you know you have a chance to win. The two weeks passed swiftly. I had an important meeting, another one with my mentor, a new job, a move to plan, and writing for this anthology. I ate healthily every day: salmon, sweet potatoes, spinach, herbal tea, no caffeine, and a progesterone injection every evening at the same time. Everything was going smoothly. My belly was starting to swell, and I felt some cramps, but no sign of blood. I held my belly in my hands, telling myself that my baby was fine, that he or she was warm and cozy, and would be born next October. I love the month of October, the inviting atmosphere it brings, and the colors of autumn. I was already thinking of ideas for celebrations we could have for him or her. One evening, my husband sat next to me in bed and said, "Can we think about names?" I burst with joy and shouted, "YES!" With a twinkle in my eye, I searched for my notes on my phone. "Oh, okay, you already started a list without telling me?" he asked, chuckling. "A little, just a few ideas. I write them down so I don't forget..."

We discussed and imagined life, as a family of three... and perhaps four in the near future. We would have liked to have three children, but with three embryos, our chances are 50% for each transfer... Hopefully the first one will be lucky. Koko doesn't believe in luck, superstitions, old wives' tales, lucky numbers, or lucky charms. He believes in science, specialized doctors, thorough research, etc. I could see that his hope was present, and he was looking forward to the day of the blood test. We didn't really talk about it to avoid putting pressure on ourselves. We knew the wind would turn very soon.

FRIDAY FEBRUARY 3, 2023

It's my grandmother Baki's celebration day in heaven. She was the one who gave me the lucky socks. It was the big day. I had a knot in my stomach and felt like vomiting from the excitement. Was it a pregnancy symptom? I managed to wait two weeks without taking a pregnancy test. I turned to Facebook groups to see conversations about the two-week wait after the transfer. The anticipation was palpable, and advice was coming from all sides. I closed the screen. I stayed positive and avoided commenting because I preferred to remain anonymous. I had two close friends, my mother, and my mother-in-law who knew, and that was already too much. The stress of telling them bad news... I was so afraid. Unable to concentrate at work, I opened my calendar, closed my calendar, opened my emails, closed my emails, checked the time... This morning, during the blood test at the clinic, the nurse confirmed that they make calls between one and one-thirty. It's one fifty-three, and still no news. I had a bad feeling. My phone rang. Private number. It was the clinic. I answered on the second ring.

"Hello?"

My voice was trembling, but I took a deep breath and tried to calm down.

"Am I speaking to Kate?"

"Yes, it's me."

"It's the nurse calling. I'm sorry to say that unfortunately, the results are negative. We'll call you back in a few weeks to meet with the doctor. She'll be able to explain the next steps. You can stop the medications and injections now."

My fingers froze and tightened around my phone. My voice broke under the weight of this news.

"Okay, thank you. I'll wait for your call. Is there anything else I can do for now?"

"No, we'll call you back soon. I'm sorry..."

I heard her helplessness at the end of the line. I thought about how she must call many women to deliver the bad news. Did she start with the positive calls? The conversation lasted a minute, not a second longer. The coldness of the call gave me goosebumps. My body leaned forward, facing the floor; I wanted to empty my guts. I was broken to the core. I was losing my first child and the will to move forward all at once... I had eaten salmon, cut out coffee, meditated, attended acupuncture appointments, slept, read, advanced my career, etc. Blame haunted me. Suddenly, I got up and dragged my feet to the bed. I had done too much. My body had anticipated this moment so much that I had created a ball of internal stress. It was my fault... My body couldn't sustain life, and my mind was my worst enemy.

Koko rushes in. "They called? It's... it's negative?" I looked at him with my haggard, glassy eyes. He had his answer.

— No, no, no, this can't be true! We're going to take a pregnancy test. It's not possible. Are you sure they said it's negative? Come on, where's the test? We'll do it to double check.

He struggled to find the pregnancy test among the papers on the table.

— Koko, forget it. It's negative. I'm not going to take a test to see the line with my own eyes.

Unable to continue speaking, I burst into tears. My anxiety took over, and my sobs turned into hiccups until there was no air in my lungs. I couldn't breathe; the room was closing in on me. I was good for nothing; my body had rejected my first baby. "Incapable" was the word that kept coming back to me as I stared at the white wall. Disconnected from the moment, Koko lay down beside me and continued to repeat, "No, this isn't true; it's impossible; I thought everything was going to work out; I thought we were going to have good news..."

Shaking his head, he didn't want to accept this defeat. He nestled into my shoulder for comfort. His wounded heart stuck to mine. I shut myself off from his outpouring of love because I was too hurt to give any in return... I felt like everything was collapsing around me. Unfortunately, I didn't think I wanted to continue in this painful and thorny ordeal. I had no idea how our couple could overcome this grief; I didn't want to hurt him anymore and drag him along on this path that had lasted three years already. He deserved to build his family, move into a big house, be with someone who would be his equal, and continue in his professional momentum. I was a burden to him, preventing him from moving forward and an embarrassment to society. His wife couldn't conceive, create life, and ensure his offspring. I hoped to be pregnant by Valentine's Day, celebrating great love.

I had two choices before me: sink into depression and disappointment or take control of myself. Start the gym again, pick up a frenetic lifestyle, and continue advancing my career. Neither of these options really appealed to me. I didn't want to continue on this train that was speeding along and preventing me from looking at the landscape. Our way of life didn't suit me anymore; how could I tell him that I had too much on my shoulders when he too was juggling too many balls?

MARCH 2023

I have to undergo a battery of tests before preparing for the next implantation. I hesitated. I revisited all the decisions made over the last decade. Unable to concentrate or sleep through the night, my brain was in turmoil and constant anxiety. My phone vibrates. My neighbor texts me: "Spinning tonight?" She's a breath of fresh air, full of enthusiasm, living her carefree single life! A ball of energy who always has wild Friday night stories. Her good mood and carefree attitude bring me to life and help me unwind. I live in the moment, listening to her latest successful dates and some that ended badly (#generationZ). She influences me in a positive way; I even started to enjoy spinning classes! I was a bit snobbish about this sport at first, but I quickly changed my mind. I'm athletic at times, but spinning was a mental hurdle I hadn't yet overcome: the neon lights, the intense music, the shouts; in short, the complete opposite of a yoga studio.

"OK, let's go!" I quickly replied.

Without thinking, I put on a sports outfit, tie up my hair, and throw my bag into the car. The car becomes my sanctuary; every time I drive, I imagine the future, organize my thoughts, and everything becomes clearer. I anticipate the vibration of the bike under my legs, the fast tempo of the music, and my cry of relief lost in the echo of the room among the other liberated women. It's a form of therapy; it's not easy, you sweat more than ever, you feel like giving up in the middle of the class because your legs are shaking, but you keep going, and in the end, you realize you were able to overcome it. Inhale, exhale. Resilience, persistence, or discipline, whatever you call it, is essential for success. When motivation stumbles, it's resilience that pushes me forward. It's my inner strength slowly growing. The ego of infertility tries to catch up with me, but I speed away under the blue and purple LED lights. Inhale. Exhale. I see the past year flash before my eyes. I increase the resistance and keep up the pace. The images fade away, replaced by a guttural cheer. I can do this.

APRIL 2023

"Every time I open social media, another pregnancy announcement pops up. I feel like I'm back in high school, like I belong to an uncool clique and the popular ones are called 'The Two Lines Crew.' They're pregnant in the blink of an eye, flaunting their joy with aesthetic beige tones and balloons revealing the baby's gender. The Two Lines Crew, I can't wait to be part of it too."

"Don't lose hope, Kate. I know it's hard to hear, but it's the truth. I didn't lose hope, and it happened."

"Yeah," I said wearily. "I'm more part of the Hardened Ovaries Crew at this stage."

Anna burst out laughing.

"You haven't lost your sense of humor!"

We gulped down our burgers in one go. I had been so careful over the past few months; no more sugar or caffeine, lots of salmon, quinoa, and blueberries, sprinkled with vegetables and beets.

"Even when I was at my lowest, I still believed. Every time, you think you've fallen into a deeper hole than before and can never climb out of it. But every time, you look up, and hope is still there."

She tenderly shared her journey towards motherhood:

"I'll always remember that Friday when the gynecologist called me to say there was a problem with my husband's semen analysis. He asked me if I wanted to talk to Pierre. No need to stress him out; besides, I don't know anything about it. We went through a series of additional tests to figure out what the problem was. It's the unknown. But here we are, success! The first time around."

"Oh yes," I said, full of hope.

Anna paused and looked out the window. I could sense a memory troubling her.

"At the six-week checkup, they tell me the heart has stopped beating."

"I'm speechless; your journey touches me so much."

"Keep hope, keep that zest for life; it will help you stay on course through the storm."

Our hands intertwined on the table, and I could feel the warmth of her support, her motherly eyes comforting me.

"Thank you for everything, Anna."

MAY 2023

The tulips slowly unfold, and spring brings a breath of fresh air. The second transfer will be this month. I will turn thirty-two this month. Strength is within me. The injections go smoothly, always with Koko's help. With each injection, he tells me a joke. Dad jokes, short and not very funny. We laugh every night; it's a ritual we'll cherish. The second transfer takes place on May 17th. On a crisp morning, I head to an acupuncture session on the same street as the clinic. I feel rested, calm, and ready to welcome the miracle within me. I let myself be guided by the music and my breath. I hold onto nothing. The notes pass through me and soothe me. I give myself a breath of hope, keeping a glimmer in my heart. I think of my mother and grandmothers, who gave life and without whom I wouldn't be here. I open my eyes as the acupuncturist removes one needle at a time, lightening my body.

"Who is the artist? This album is enchanting."

"The talented Alexandra Stréliski."

Some moments will always be etched in our memory due to our attachment to a smell, a touch, or even a song. Alexandra Stréliski reminds me of my serene state just before my second transfer. A perfect 5AA baby. The transfer was more about openness and acceptance than the first one. The fear had dissipated, and the joy of carrying life had settled in. I then took a break from several responsibilities to give my body and mind a well-deserved rest, accompanied by meditation, conversations with my mother in the spa, the kindness of Koko, and the gentleness I showed myself. There it is. I feel it. It's the right time, the right month, and above all, the right mindset.

MAY 26, 2023

The day before my thirty-second birthday, I received the call. Koko and I take a little break in bed in the middle of the day. We kiss, we laugh, and we keep an eye on my phone nearby. The phone rings.

Certainly, one should only have one love in this world,
One love, just one, however whimsical it may be;
And I who search for it thus, noble and subtle,
Find that it is to my soul a deep wound.

—*EMILE NELLIGAN*

The pain was so deep that my numb body did not feel the destruction of my happiness. Koko meets my senseless gaze. He takes my hand and feels my tremors. The tears don't flow. I slowly come back to my senses and hear his distant words telling me not to worry. He chooses his words carefully, as his hope dissipates. I catch it and put a hand on his heart:

"It's just an obstacle. Let's keep on going, keep on pushing through."

Stréliski's piano notes soothe me. The soft chords resonate within me, dissipating my turmoil. Just as in the variations of her compositions, my emotions dance between contrasts.

MAY 27, 2023

Amidst the cheerful "Happy birthday" wishes, I open my eyes to a huge chocolate cake with a candle in the middle. This scene of love gives me a surge of stoicism. Tears roll down my cheeks as I blow out the candle. My wish, it is written in these pages, felt through Koko's tenderness, it is palpable and so close.

I will be a mother one day, and until that day, I will live every moment of my life with passion and boldness. Life doesn't stop here, not today, not tomorrow. I write these words to soothe and inspire women on fertility journeys, but above all, to offer my future child all the courage in the world. They will know that obstacles and defeats are an integral part of life. We must know how to dance on rainy days to find beauty. To scream at the top of our lungs in a spinning class or a concert, to express the passion burning within us. To embrace loved ones with an emotion so deep that words are almost irrelevant. I promise myself, as I blow out this candle, to turn every challenge into a lesson of resilience, every detour into an unexpected opportunity, and every tear into a pearl of wisdom. With every sunrise, I will rise with determination, ready to embrace the beauty of each new day. I will marvel at the flowers blooming, the laughter echoing, and the kisses sealing precious moments. I will create memories that gently settle into the corners of my soul, forming a timeless treasure.

And when the day comes when I have the honor of becoming a mother, I will impart to my child the strength to persevere, to dream without limits, and to marvel at the magic of life. I will be there to encourage them to pursue their passions. I will be the pillar upon which my child can lean, a comforting presence amidst the tumults of destiny. I will urge them to embrace their own trials and to find the hidden beauty in every challenge. Thus, I will conclude this chapter by turning the page towards the future, embracing every line of my destiny. Life, like a symphony, will continue to play its melodious and sometimes discordant notes. And I will be there, ready to pedal to the rhythm of each measure, savoring every moment of happiness and writing my own love story with life.

A conclusion that will never truly be an end, but rather a suspension point, a promise of infinite continuity, where love and science will one day create my little miracle.

This is only the beginning of our story.

CHAPTER 2

I'M NOT MADE OF GLASS

By Andrée-Anne Charron

I'm a 5'10" woman. High school Ethics teacher. Yoga instructor. Traveler. In psychotherapy for the past 15 years.

JUNE 2022

In a room with plastic vertical blinds and four blue walls, pale and dull, my thighs stick to the plastic chair. I grip underneath it to restrain the restlessness of my legs. After taking my blood pressure for a second time, my family doctor consults her computer and reviews her notes. These moments always seem longer when waiting and fearing the worst. To avoid thinking about it, I focus on what is around me, down to the smallest details. I'm used to it; in the past year, I've visited more medical clinics than new cities according to the report Google Map sends me by email each month. My eyes dart around in search of anything and everything: a black mousepad, a notepad, a nearly empty brochure dispenser with one of them reading, "STBBI's: Understanding them, Avoiding them". The wait gives rise to numerous observations regarding the decor and lack of vitality in these establishments, despite their dedication to health.

"You're experiencing post-traumatic stress. It's not uncommon for this to happen after a traumatic event like the one you just went through.

Last April, I had to be hospitalized and undergo emergency surgery after four days of pelvic pain. I had peritonitis, which is an infection of the peritoneum, the membrane that covers the abdominal walls. The exact cause remains unknown. During my painful hospital stay, I caught COVID-19 and developed C. Difficile infection. Yes, I bought a lottery ticket. No, I didn't win!

Post-traumatic stress. These three words play on repeat in my head. When I got home, I took a shower to assimilate the news and let the tension of that appointment drain away. I always thought this diagnosis was reserved for war veterans and immigrant children who have experienced war... As I think back on the events of the past few months, I've come to accept it: spending four days in the emergency room with sharp pain in my lower abdomen and coming out of the hospital with a hunched back and a long scar on my abdomen; seeing my daily life completely disrupted, unable to finish the school year with my students; waking up in the middle of the night and, come morning, feeling an existential dread gripping me to my core. As the water flows, I realize that the past two months in recovery have been anxiety-induced, but in reality, I've been battling this feeling of powerlessness for two years. It's been two years since I've felt like I'm fighting against myself, waging war on my body."

As I stepped out of the shower, I cried. I cried because of the hospital stay, but also because of the past two years: the COVID-19 pandemic, the loneliness, the powerlessness, the setbacks, the infertility... Two years of negative pregnancy tests; of waiting and hypervigilance at the slightest sign of pregnancy; of taking hormones, ovulation tests, and appointments where I have to go alone because of COVID-19; of nightmares where I wake up in the middle of the night, gasping for air. Two years of holding my breath when someone tells me, "I have good news to tell you."

I can't breathe anymore.

THE BEGINNING

JULY 2019

For my boyfriend Maxime and I, the baby project began in the heat of summer in the Algarve. As soon as we arrived at our rental in a charming fishing village, we wasted no time. We were eager and excited for the start of this new adventure! A few days later, crossing the Strait of Gibraltar, we attended the wedding of one of my friends in Morocco. My partner in crime for trips to the dollar store between classes, during our teaching degree, to buy candies and survive the long hours of training. We had formed friendships with other girls in our final year, and we dreamed of traveling together after our university studies. With four years of experience under our belt, some savings, and the summer off, the timing was perfect for this trip and, by extension, to start trying to conceive a child.

As we soaked up the sun among girls, in the desert of a North African village, I raised the subject:

— Hey, Maxime and I made the decision before leaving, not to pack any condoms.

— Really? Us too!

— It would be so exotic to tell our children they were conceived in Africa.

— Definitely!

Upon our return from the trip, within a few months of each other, my friends, one by one, learned they were pregnant. With a hint of envy, I was happy for them. Deep down, my concerns about not succeeding were skyrocketing. Even though it took longer for one of them and we were able to discuss this endless wait on several occasions, I quickly felt alone in this fertility journey.

As the months passed, I began to suspect that something wasn't right. The reality is, I've suffered from intense menstrual cramps since my first period. As a teenager, unable to attend school on the first day of my cycle, I had consulted a doctor who told me it was normal to feel pain during periods. I had left the doctor's office without overthinking the matter, a prescription for birth control pills in hand. I took it for over ten years. However, a few months into our baby-making process, I realized the pain had slowly returned, getting stronger every month. Waking up in the middle of the night, nauseous from the pain, I wanted to rip out my ovaries. I began to wonder if it was normal to be this sick during my periods. At a follow-up visit with my family doctor a few months after our return from the trip, I mentioned it to her. She prescribed painkillers, reassuring me that there was nothing to worry about for now: fertility referrals are made after a year of trying when you are under 35.

NOVEMBER 2020

On the day before my 30th birthday, I received a phone call informing me that we are part of the statistics of one in six couples suffering from infertility. Yes, by phone, you read that correctly. It would have been a little less awful on Zoom. Initial diagnosis: polycystic ovaries. In retrospect, I realize they had to open my abdomen to discover my endometriosis, a diagnosis that takes an average of 7 to 10 years to obtain and affects 1 in 10 women. The silver lining: my peritonitis allowed me to receive an official diagnosis!

At that moment, we are presented with the option of trying naturally with a little hormonal boost or start inseminations. We opt for the first option, excited at the prospect of maybe having twins (8% chance according to the doctor). Completely shaken by this phone call where I blanked out any information after the fertility doctor mentioned "polycystic ovaries," but excited about this fresh start, I am also relieved that they found the cause of a year of unsuccessful attempts and unbearable pain during my periods. At least, that's what I thought at the time...

Before starting the medication and hormonal pills, I have to get blood tests done again. With services reduced due to the pandemic, I have the choice of paying $1000 at a private clinic or skip them altogether. I discussed it with my sister, who is a nurse, hoping she can do the blood tests at home. The only catch is that we are in the midst of a pandemic (access to the hospital is prohibited for visitors) and she has to quickly transport the vials to work for analysis. Hoping she wouldn't have mandatory overtime that morning, I met her in the hospital parking lot where she draws my blood in the car after her night shift. At –30 degrees Celsius, the heated seats aren't enough to warm my frozen veins; filling the 15 vials is not an easy task! On the way back home, we talked on the phone, each in our own car, about the possibility of me eventually giving birth at the hospital where she works. I imagine myself pregnant, with my sister by my side, to remind me to breathe during labor.

No matter how much I imagine giving birth, with my sister at my bedside, the months go by, one after another: positive ovulation tests, negative pregnancy tests. I realize that fertility is a matter of luck and not merit. Despite my efforts to stay positive, manage stress, exercise, reduce alcohol, and eat well, I still haven't been rewarded. At the end of each month, I'm broken-hearted, as if I have been left behind. I listened to Michael Kiwanuka's song "Cold Little Heart" on repeat:

> Did you ever want it?
> Did you want it bad?
> Oh my, it tears me apart.

Fairly early in the process, I tried to connect with people who are or have experienced infertility. In my inner circle, except for a coworker, no one has undergone fertility treatments. A support group like AA, but for infertile women must exist, right? I started researching online. My parents were long-time members of Compassionate Friends, a group for those who have faced the death of a child. I want, like them, to be able to share my fears, concerns, and sorrows with others who are going through the same experiences as me. Apart from a Facebook group, I find nothing similar. Discouraged, I remember that the sister of my friend, the one who got married in Morocco, had two children through in vitro fertilization.

I asked her if she would be willing to answer my questions. She agrees.

I found my "fertility buddy."

JUNE 2021

My first insemination takes place at the end of my school year. Exhausted but excited, I stopped at the local landmark fast food joint, right next to the fertility clinic, because I need to have a full bladder for the procedure. In the waiting room, I sip my orange juice while my "fertility buddy" and I chat. I'm so happy she's accompanying me for that first time!

The wait is long, and I start to regret getting the large orange juice. I REALLY NEED TO PEE!!! Fortunately, the procedure only lasts two minutes, and I rush to the bathroom as soon as my appointment is over. With a good sperm analysis and fireworks in the evening for our national holiday, the stars seemed aligned to have our first positive test.

Exactly 14 days later, I have to send the result of my pregnancy test to the clinic. I take it while camping up north, in the woods at 4 a.m. Unable to fall back asleep due to excitement, I impatiently wait for a reasonable hour to get up. Squatting in the damp woods with the test in one hand and the flashlight in the other, I tell myself it would make a great story to tell if it was positive. Wrapped in my sleeping bag, the 3-minute wait feels endless.

Negative.

While reminding ourselves that it doesn't always work on the first try, Maxime and I walk that morning to the statue of the Virgin Mary at the top of the fjord. During the hike, this first setback continues to occupy my thoughts. If only I could get pregnant as easily as the Virgin Mary!! I hope this is a sign... Maybe if I pray really REALLY hard to the baby Jesus, the next insemination will be the one.

FALL 2021

I reluctantly go to the clinic and wait for my name to be called. I try not to feed my flood of negative thoughts, but it's hard. To do this, I focus on what's around me: a picture of the Biosphere on the wall, a secretary overwhelmed with calls about the free IVF program, women, alone, on their phones, all here for the same reason, the desire to have a child.

On my part, I prefer not to spend time on social media. Watching high school acquaintances throw pink or blue powder in their faces at their gender reveal party, I don't need that. I understand that others' happiness doesn't diminish mine, but it's still difficult to be constantly confronted with what you desire most. Lately, every time we see our friends, one of them announces the arrival of their first, second, or third child. The feeling of injustice grows, especially when I'm told "What is meant to be will be" after mustering all my courage to talk about my infertility. Some good "pop psychology" just to rub salt in the wound. That or the famous example of the friend everyone knows who got pregnant naturally while waiting for fertility treatments or after a pregnancy. It's because "sometimes we want too much, we stress too much about it, right?" Thanks to our Catholic heritage for this zero guilt-tripping advice. We all know that friend who won the "baby lottery." I may hope for the best, but if I'm under the care of a medical team, it's because I'm realistic and my chances of conceiving naturally are low with or without stress. "But, you know, worst-case scenario, there's always adoption." Yes, but no. If Maxime and I had wanted to adopt, honestly, we would have chosen that path long before assisted reproduction. My justification is well rehearsed now when this option is thrown at me, which seems so simple in the eyes of those who easily conceive naturally.

— Madame Charron, it's your turn.

I enter a small white room and sit on the examination table. I notice a photograph on the wall of a hand holding white and brown eggs. I cling to this image until the doctor enters and tells me, before proceeding with my insemination, that the results of the sperm analysis are not very encouraging. I burst into tears as soon as he closed the door to the room. I am devastated. I don't even want to get up from the examination table.

The sixth insemination will be another failure.

HYMN TO SPRING

APRIL 2022

Enrolled on the waiting list for IVF for a few months, Maxime and I were on a mandatory treatment break. This is when the accumulated fatigue from past inseminations hit me. My ovulation was extremely painful this month, my back hurt badly. I now know it's due to endometriosis. Thanks to the most experienced doctor at my new fertility clinic who saw the endometrioma on one of my recent ultrasounds and finally acknowledged my pain. Despite the relief it brought me, I couldn't bear to suffer anymore. At that moment, completely discouraged, I kept repeating to myself that I wished for a hysterectomy once the "baby project" was either realized or buried forever.

One Saturday afternoon, I received a call from my little sister announcing her pregnancy. I suspected it was coming, and I had already mentioned to her in conversation that a surprise pregnancy announcement at a gathering would be difficult for me, that I preferred to manage my emotions first on my own, in order to then be able to take an interest in her maternity journey. Otherwise, I find myself frozen, holding back my tears and thoughts that constantly bring me back to my own reality. I've experienced it too often. This feeling even led me to avoid certain dinners with friends or to anticipate the announcement of a pregnancy, as if to protect myself from a life's mishap that I can't control. My sister shares her happiness with delicacy and empathy. We cry with joy, with sadness, we confide in each other, we laugh. With this news in mind, the next day, I make an effort to leave my house and visit the Museum of Fine Arts. I am determined to stay happy and not to dwell on my own failures.

It's the following Saturday that I suddenly returned to the hospital for acute pain in the lower abdomen.

Time stood still.

The day after the surgery, the sixty-year-old surgeon, a little rough on the edges, came to see me.

"You had peritonitis. Originally, you had a pelvic infection, that's what they diagnosed you with in the emergency room. The infection was spread throughout your peritoneum and abdomen, even in your small intestine and stomach. I cleaned it all up for you," he said, making sweeping gestures with his arms toward my abdomen. "Your Fallopian tubes and ovaries were swollen. You have some cysts on your ovaries because of your endometriosis. I called the gynecologist, who was delivering a baby, to come and see this."

As the surgeon described the horror of my suffering over the past few days, no words could come out of my mouth.

"Listen, you had endometriosis tissue on your appendix. I removed it to make sure we wouldn't have to reoperate on you for that in a few days. The infection is gone. Everything has been cleaned up. But your endometriosis, listen carefully here, it's quite severe. A lot of swelling around the uterus. Anyway, if I hadn't known you were trying to conceive, I would have removed everything," he said firmly.

A tear quickly slid down my cheek. From that point on, I couldn't hear anything anymore. Lying in a hospital bed, immobilized by the pain in my stomach and by two catheters, one connected to my stomach and the other to my bladder, I felt like a truck had just hit me.

"It's not time to cry. You need to get better so you can start walking again and get out of here."

His words hit me like a slap in the face, but it was with hindsight that I understood that I needed that tough love not to dwell on my fate. In the following days, even though I tried not to think about it, tried to get better and get out of the hospital, everything around me reminded me of the desire to have a child and the surgeon's harsh words.

Remove everything.

As my hospital neighbor left the room we shared, the curtain separating us allowed a glimpse of daylight. I hadn't seen daylight for almost a week. I spotted a large tree in the middle of the hospital courtyard. Its branches were covered with small buds. I started to cry when I realized I had missed this fabulous moment when the trees bloom in spring. I discovered an obsession with seedlings last year. Facing infertility, watching a seed germinate and blossom in my garden gives me great satisfaction. Seeing some seeds germinate while others don't, gives me a certain sense of control over a phenomenon I can't control within myself. Within the hospital walls, deprived of internet connection, I listened repeatedly to the album by Pierre Lapointe that I had downloaded on my phone for my museum visit, especially his cover of Félix Leclerc's "Hymne Au Printemps":

Vois, les fleurs ont recommencé
Dans l'étable crient les nouveau-nés
Viens voir la vieille barrière rouillée
Endimanchée de toiles d'araignée [2]

During my recovery at home, listening to this song and watching life go on outside my window, I often wondered why the surgeon didn't remove everything: all the suffering that comes with this wretched reproductive system and the uncertainty that haunts me every day since. Singing these gentle words repeatedly brought me a gust of hope and freedom like the promise of a new spring.

In my mind, to get through these difficult months, I needed a break. The waiting and not knowing if I could ever bear a child drained me emotionally. I completely let go. After all I had been through, I wanted to enjoy life, travel, and have a good time with my partner, without living in the limbo we had been in for three years. We went to Western Canada that summer with my parents, and I thought that could be the rest of our lives: trips, dinners with family and friends, museum outings, yoga and spinning classes whenever I wanted. Even though this freedom and independence was inviting, when I think of a life without a

---

2 Look, the flowers have started again
In the stable, the newborns cry
Come see the old rusty gate
Dressed up in cobwebs

child, I feel a little pinch in my heart. I never dreamed of being a mother, but I would really like to experience motherhood. I felt this desire later in my twenties, when I met my boyfriend. We shared the same values and the aspiration to grow together in a serious relationship. From the first months of our life together, seeing him entertain his friends' children, I immediately saw in him that he would make a great dad. Since then, the idea of seeing a little bit of us make its way in life has only grown stronger.

But faced with the surgeon's unsettling words, it was easier for me to give up the project. Maxime didn't understand how I could be so affected by the uncertainty. That's just who I am: either fully committed or not at all. On the journey back from an appointment, where I had my staples removed, I recall confiding in my dad about grieving over our baby project. Seated in the car, at a red light, his voice trembled with emotion as he responded, 'Life is a succession of losses, both minor and major."

FALL 2022

In a dark and uninviting room, I meet a new gynecologist four months after my ordeal for a first postoperative follow-up. I'm surprised by her response regarding the continuation of the baby project.

— Go for it, it's time to resume fertility treatments while you're still young.

She makes me realize that I experienced a streak of bad luck this spring. SHIT HAPPENS.

— Could peritonitis have affected the success of an IVF?

— No, not at all. However, it's possible that you may need surgery if your tubes are damaged. It would be a day surgery where we would make four small incisions in the abdomen to remove the tubes through the navel. Nothing as invasive as what you experienced.

— So, I would become infertile?

— Yes, but it could give you better chances of success. Currently, you still have a one in three chance of IVF working the first time.

I'm a little unsettled by her optimism and disconcerted by her confidence, but she gives me the courage to contact my fertility clinic again. The baby project is revived.

I'm scheduled for an ultrasound a month later, and even though my ovarian reserve went from good in 2020 to adequate, the doctor says I shouldn't need surgery for the moment. All in all, good news! No surgery. And an adequate ovarian reserve isn't bad. I accept the situation, even though I want to understand how I could lose so many eggs in two years. Is this the normal course of life? I knew that gradually, women become less fertile, but I didn't think it would lower me by one notch. That's fine, OK? CORRECT. Anyway, you know what they say, it only takes one for it to work (but objectively, I'd like to have more than one, please). Please? Who do I ask? The universe? The goddess of fertility? Baby Jesus? Maybe if I had continued my Sunday classes, this whole process would be easier. How do I explain that my reserve went from good to adequate? It's part of GOD'S PLAN. Would it be easier to accept that way?

Maxime and I still decide to enjoy the last few months of 2022 before diving into IVF. My mental health is good, the stress of post-traumatic shock is behind me. I don't want to lose my balance right away.

THE BEGINNING, TAKE 2

JANUARY 2023

A week before starting the injections, I'm already anticipating the side effects and possible complications. What if I get hyper stimulated? What if the infection reappears? What if I don't respond well to the stimulation? What if I end up in the hospital, yet again? What if we're doing all this for nothing? I'm aware that it's a process with no guarantees. I'm not even on the hormones yet and I'm already getting on my nerves (and my partner's!). And when I experience an anxiety episode, everything becomes a source of stress.

As far back as I can remember, anxiety has always been part of my life. During school, I couldn't fall asleep the night before an exam or a presentation. I remember, as a child, going downstairs to join my parents who were watching television. My mother would make room for me on the couch, and I would watch late-night talk shows with them. I know that blue light is to be avoided when dealing with insomnia, but for me, there's a comforting memory in watching television when my endometriosis pains wake me up in the middle of the night on the first day of my period. I indulge on two anti-inflammatory tablets, while eating a peanut butter toast. Heating pad on my stomach, legs in a butterfly position in front of an episode of The Office, I wait until the pain slowly fades away and sleep takes over.

After a two-week holiday break, I return to work feeling wiped out. I'm drained from my vacation. Drained from seeing too many people and planning too many activities to avoid anxiety *#livingwithanxiety*. Furthermore, I have to stop taking the contraceptive pill that was prescribed to me after my surgery and start hormone injections in six days. The cramps are back, so is the pain. And the headaches… *#livingwithendometriosis*. Yeah!

One Saturday afternoon, I'm tempted to Google my abdominal discomfort for the thousandth time. All medical searches being now forbidden by my family doctor, I mustered up the courage to get up from the couch and go outside. Breathing in the fresh air helps me find my center. It feels like my ovaries are pulling my belly down to the ground, but keeping active draws my attention elsewhere. Everything passes.

I like to remember the words a hospital attendant told me on a sleepless night when I was looking for answers to everything happening to me, raging against injustice. I take deep breaths; the thoughts slowly dissipate. Will taking hormones worsen the pain? I don't know if I can bear that for long. I look around me; the fir trees are beautiful with their coats of glistening snow. I sit on a bench in the middle of the park. As I gaze at the clouds, a thought resurfaces: how far does this desire to have children go? As I stare at the sky, tears well up in my eyes.

The white clouds drift swiftly across the pure blue sky, mirroring the pace of my racing thoughts. Today, they seem to hurry along, much like my restless mind. Lost in my thoughts, I often overlook the constant presence of the serene blue backdrop. The tranquility I've been seeking has always surrounded me, patiently waiting to be acknowledged.

As I resume my walk, I am determined not to let anxiety overcome me. But how can I experience the IVF more serenely? Last spring, my mother asked me if I was thankful the antibiotics cured me. Feeling gratitude in one of the worst moments of my life seemed absurd to me. However, I started doing it when my doctor prescribed lorazepam for my anxiety attacks, and I was afraid of becoming addicted because the label said in big letters "MAY CAUSE DEPENDENCY". That was enough to make me anxious about taking my anxiety medication. Saying "thank you" added an extra awareness to my action, like a promise to myself: "Thank you for allowing me to fall asleep quickly, I won't make a habit of it." When I returned from my walk, I wrote on a sticky note "Grateful for these injections to give us a chance for a baby," and I stuck it on the Ziploc bag filled with syringes that the pharmacist gave me.

A few days later, I started the injections. I had already done a few for the inseminations, but this time, I have to mix medications, adding an extra challenge. In a panic, I called my sister on video chat.

— HELP, I don't understand how to draw all the liquid with the syringe.

My sister, folding laundry for her newborn baby, looks at the equipment I have in my hands.

— They didn't give you a larger syringe? Otherwise, you'll have to repeat the process several times because the liquid won't fit completely in that one.

I rummage through the Ziploc bag filled with syringes. There was a bigger one! In the stress of the moment, I hadn't seen it. Since the beginning of the call, Maxime has been holding my phone to film me, so my sister can supervise my back and forth between the two vials. When the mixture is done, I switch syringes and fill it with the necessary dose. My sister explains that I have to flick the syringe and pull the plunger slightly down then up to remove air bubbles. A few drops fly onto Maxime's face.

— Watch what you're doing, I got some in my eye!

— Oh noooo, I hope you don't end up with an egg growing in your eye! Go rinse quickly!

I'm trembling inside, but everything's fine. I disinfect my belly and I'm ready for the injection.

3, 2, 1, go! I wasn't ready, I start over. 3, 2, 1, GO!

I press the plunger. It's done! Proud of myself, I thank my sister again.

It was like a little remote nursing class!

— Put the needle in the disposal bin, you stress me out by continuing to talk with the syringe in your hands!

The next day, it's my sister-in-law who accompanies me for my second injection between the main course and dessert service.

She has already taken a class to become a nursing assistant, which reassures me. Evening activities certainly make managing hormone intake a bit more complicated, but they allow me to take my mind off things and avoid falling into hypervigilance.

On our way to my first ultrasound, my partner finds me silent. He knows I'm nervous. For the first time since we started fertility treatment, he'll be able to accompany me at every step of the process. His presence comforts me, especially when I'm on the examination table waiting for the doctor. When the doctor finally arrives, he measures the follicles he sees on the left ovary and leaves the probe in my vagina before checking on the right. I tense up with discomfort and wonder what he'll say to break the seemingly endless silence.

— You're responding very well to ovarian stimulation; you have 8 follicles on each side.

I feel relieved. Before leaving the room, I start to cry. The best-case scenario has unfolded. Following the preparatory IVF videos, Maxime and I have been enthusiastically discussing the hopes for the egg retrieval: 15 perfect follicles. In all the scenarios presented, that was the best since the follicles not only need to be mature but also of good quality to continue developing after fertilization. A large number of follicles is not synonymous with quality.

Then, two days later, came my second ultrasound. The young gynecologist gently inserts the probe. (Thank you!) Already, he deserves 5 stars on Google for his friendly demeanor and sensitivity during the procedure. His gentleness and optimism remind me of some previous painful and cold examinations where you really feel like just a number in the medical system. As he navigates gently inside my uterus, he notes the damage from the storm of last spring. Making his way through the debris of my endometriosis, his eyes light up when he finally comes across the treasure chest filled with follicles.

— I'm very pleased to see what I'm seeing! 15 beautiful and uniform follicles. You're responding really well to ovarian stimulation.

My partner and I are so happy, he can clearly see our huge smiles behind our masks and the emotion in my eyes. We take every little victory we can in this process. Ovulation will be triggered tomorrow and the egg retrieval will take place two days later. The embryo transfer will have to wait for a cycle since I'm at risk of ovarian hyperstimulation. The gynecologist reassures me by prescribing medication for it and informs us that the blastocysts will be stored in the freezer until everything settles down. To think that I was so afraid of ovarian hyperstimulation. Everything is under control!

Pure coincidence or a sign from destiny, a picture representing the Algarve is in the recovery room after my egg retrieval. I like to believe that there is magic in this whole process; let's remember that it was in the Algarve that Maxime and I started our baby project almost four years ago. The sedatives they administered left me in a moment of unconsciousness. I hear the nurse say from afar that a total of 19 eggs were retrieved. Of this number, 13 are mature and fertilized. On day 1, we have 7 blastocysts. I'm a bit disappointed to learn that about half didn't fuse, but I was told that it was to be expected. After all, on a blind date, it doesn't always click on the first try. I figure my eggs must be as picky as myself, when I was on the dating scene. When a friend wanted to introduce me to Maxime seven years ago, I refused when I found out he wasn't over 6 feet tall. A few months later, we hit it off at a party she invited me to, without telling me he would be there, and we exchanged numbers.

Day 2, still 7 blastocysts! I'm on cloud nine, they've all held up. To avoid falling into anxiety, I dive into a DIY project to pass the time. I drop acrylic paint droplets onto paper to represent cells and cut them out to form seven beautiful, more or less perfect circles. Knowing that the natural selection process will take place and that we'll lose about half of them, I represent some blastocysts with fewer cells. Days go by, and I think of them each time I glance at my craft project. I hope they're developing well. I'm starting to grow attached to them even though I know they're not babies. They're so beautiful that I could turn them into artwork. Crafting and working keep my mind occupied because I find the time long before the embryologist's call. I feel like a child counting down the sleep until Christmas.

The day before the call, I started experiencing back pain and more frequent cramps in the lower abdomen. These symptoms bring back bad memories. All day, I battle against my anxiety. To calm myself, I call the nurse who reminds me that my period will come in the next few days. Feeling nauseous and bloated due to hyperstimulation, I put all my hopes into the embryologist's call, hoping it will be worth it.

The next day, she informs us that five are still in the race but aren't yet mature enough. They'll be left in the incubators for an additional 24 hours to continue developing. I don't know if it's good news or not. I sleep poorly that night, thinking about my five blastocysts. It's in the morning that we receive news: only one embryo will be frozen.

As I hang up, tears stream down my face. I was certain we'd have two, maybe three if we were lucky enough. Just one embryo means zero backup if it doesn't implant; we'd have to start all over again. It's a lot of pressure for just one embryo. Even though I'm frustrated with life, my eternal optimist consoles me and reminds me that it's the strongest one of all, that it's the right one. While my anxiety is already considering a plan B, eventually resorting to egg donation if this transfer doesn't work, Maxime brings me back to reality. One step at a time, he repeats.

That's why I love him. He's realistic, down-to-earth, calm, and pragmatic. Everything I'm not. I wipe away my tears and rush to open social media in search of positive stories with a single embryo in the fertility group. There are plenty. Our own story, I still don't know how it ends.

MARCH 2023

It's in a Montreal café near Maxime's office that I pass the time before the transfer of our embryo. Whether it sticks or not, I feel like I'm creating memories that will be forever etched in my mind. Making the most of it. After all, who can say they had the chance to see their embryo on a giant screen before it embarked on its journey into the uterine cavity? A fun adventure.

Even though the past few years haven't always been fun, there has been beauty in all of it. Most importantly, there's still hope. To find happiness, I've learned to see beyond the misfortunes. To see love in the little things. Like Maxime's grandmother who gave me a small medal of a saint whose name I can't remember and who prays for us every day. Like the support of my friends who I can rely on to eat fries together after my transfer, to bring me luck.

Like the pride I feel in my role as an aunt to my sister's baby and godmother to my sister-in-law's daughter: the joy of buying them cute outfits, telling them stories, making them smile, the chance to rock them to sleep, feeling their little bodies breathe in my arms, or getting vomit in my hair after a feed. One day, they'll understand how much I love them. I've always had a great propensity for happiness. All my childhood, my mother told me I was her little ray of sunshine. One day, I was that embryo in the darkness, growing in her womb to make my place in this world. While she cried the death of her second child, I fought, I clung on.

Life, so mysterious, so fragile. We take it for granted. I'm thankful for the progress of science and all the medical staff who treated me in the past two years, allowing me to see my embryo on the screen today. But above all, thanks to Maxime. My love. My part-time caregiver. My beacon. During the long wait after the transfer, intrusive thoughts gave way to nursery rhymes for big kids. In the car, in the shower, doing the dishes, I repeated these words like a broken record:

On va changer d'air pour vrai mon p'tit cœur
T'es mieux de te tenir prêt.
Je suis pas faite en chocolat.
On n'est pas fait en chocolat.

—*TRICOT MACHINE*[3]

APRIL 2023

It's been so long since I've been to my favorite yoga studio. In the mountain pose, where you simply stand, arms by your side and palms facing forward, my body sways like a pendulum. My toes gripping the ground desperately try not to let me fall. I relax my knees and try to distribute the weight by anchoring the soles of my feet to the ground. Connected to my mat, I rediscover my strength and stability, despite the strong winds of the past few days. What joy to find myself again. It's as if I forgot to be in my body during the marathon of medications, blood draws, and phone calls of the past few days. Today, I slowly learn to trust it again, to continue to believe that it will one day carry life. In the center of my mat, while the teacher speaks, I remember my

3 We're going to change the scenery for real, baby.
You better get ready.
I'm not made of chocolate.
We're not made of chocolate.
—*Tricot machine*

dream from last night: another embryo had been transferred to me. I was carrying it inside me and caressing my belly. It felt so real. Since I received the call from the nurse telling me that our only embryo had stopped developing, I realize for the first time that it's no longer inside me. After nesting there for a few days, it's gone. Still standing on my mat, as I exhale deeply, I feel a great emptiness in the depths of my belly.

> « Elle dit que c'est un oiseau
> envolé de sa cage.
> Elle dit que c'est la cage
> qui la fait pleurer.
> Le vide laissé par l'oiseau
> Le vent qui traverse la cage
> Le vent,
> ça mouille les yeux. »
>
> —LES SOEURS BOULAY[4]

4 "She says it's a bird
flying away from its cage.
She says it's the cage
that makes her cry.
The emptiness left by the bird
The wind that passes through the cage
The wind,
it makes the eyes wet."
—*Les soeurs Boulay*

CHAPTER 3

THE LOSS

BY Sasha Plante

> *At the temple, there is a poem called 'Loss' carved into the stone. It has three words, but the poet has scratched them out. You cannot read loss, you can only feel it.".*
>
> —*MEMOIRS OF A GEISHA*, ARTHUR GOLDEN

In this chapter, I take you into the heart of my diary. You will witness the hardest and most beautiful moments of my life. I hope to move, inform, and comfort all those who read me.

I was hired as an orderly a few months ago. I redirected my career to be even closer to patients, or residents in my case, as I work in a long-term care facility. My academic setback to become a licensed practical nurse affected my morale and, in the process, destroyed the relationship I was in. The stars must have been aligned though, because I found a job I loved. I've never enjoyed life this much, especially in the company of my friends, and, believe it or not, I met someone! Like me, he is an orderly. A bit older, handsome, funny, and he helped me a lot at work. We developed an exceptional bond. There were dates, a trip, my move to his place, engagement, and even though he had a vasectomy a year before meeting me, we both wanted a child. I had several serious relationships over the years, and in those relationships of trust and love, there came a time when protection was set aside. Yet, there was never a pregnancy. And as some of my friends got pregnant despite condoms and IUDs, I began to doubt my ability to have children.

Who doesn't recall the famous wooden penis used by the nurse to explain how to properly unroll a condom? How everyone was excited during the distribution of a few dozen small red packets, even though no one really understood the menstrual cycle. We all knew that a little pill could be a contraceptive method, but what is a fallopian tube? And what's the connection between STIs and fertility? Of course, I had no idea that 10 years after starting to be sexually active, an old asymptomatic chlamydia would be the cause of the hardest chapter of my life: infertility.

JULY 13, 2021

It's been a long time since I've kept a journal. When I was young, I would write about my misfortunes and hope they would go away by closing the journal. This one is a little different because it will allow you to know where you come from and also how much you were wanted. You must know that we have already come a long way. To begin with, there are my fertility tests that I took a while ago. According to my doctor, everything was normal. So, if I have never been pregnant, it would be either the incompatibility or my weight. She says I am underweight, but I've seen smaller women than me get pregnant so I'm in doubt. 114.2 pounds, not so bad. Stef had his vasectomy reversal, and immediately after the surgery, there were already sperm. That was encouraging! We are waiting for my doctor to receive the results of the semen analysis, and in the meantime, we are doing "home trials." We monitor when I ovulate, and every month, we fear the day when my period is due to arrive. It's always a disappointment when it happens, but we don't lose hope.

JULY 14, 2021

I got my period last night. Another attempt fails! At last, I'm scheduled for a few check ups. On August 31, we're scheduled for an appointment with my doctor at the fertility clinic. I will talk to her about insemination because clearly, there is something wrong with me. Soon, we will know, and I am eager to have a POSITIVE result.

"I'm not on the pill, but don't worry, I can't have children!" That's what I said to my previous boyfriend. It's also that phrase that led me to consult at a fertility clinic. At first, you don't understand anything, and you're sent for unpronounceable tests that you didn't even know existed. You feel like they're looking for cancer. They draw dozens of tubes of blood from me; they test my urine; they take samples from my cervix, perform endovaginal radiographs; they inject liquid into my uterus using a probe while I lie under a huge machine. In short, I'm asked to lift my legs high and bring my buttocks closer together. However, I was far from imagining that the blood, the needles, the legs up in the air, and even the operating room were just the beginning. At this stage, you start doing research, still hoping that pregnancy will happen somewhat like everyone else's, as a beautiful surprise.

AUGUST 5, 2021

Still no sign of you in my belly. It's been a while since I wrote, but there's nothing new, really. We went back to work after two weeks of vacation, and we are still waiting for the results of the semen analysis. We're both impatient! Stef marked on the calendar the day I'm supposed to have my period. On my end, I think about this friend who is going to have her second child, about another friend who just had her first, and about my best friend who just removed her IUD to get pregnant. I can't wait for the next appointment to ask my doctor about insemination. Fingers crossed, she says yes!

AUGUST 16, 2021

Today, I received a call from my fertility clinic to confirm my appointment on August 31. The nurse sent me requests for blood tests for both Stef and I by email. He will go for his on Thursday, and for me, it will be next month since it needs to be done between the first and fifth day of my menstrual cycle. Good news, she got the result of the semen analysis and will give us the results at the appointment! I'm excited! I can't stop watching what the insemination procedure is like, and God knows I can't wait to have you in my belly!

SEPTEMBER 1, 2021

Such good news! Yesterday, I finally received the phone call I was waiting for. The doctor authorized me to start treatments for insemination because all the tests I did were clear. The semen analysis results were perfect. I'm so happy, and I want everything to happen right now. I still have one blood test to do and I'll also have time to do my Pap test. I will start the process in October, when I get my period. Another step forward! There's a one in ten chance of having a multiple pregnancy. I did the famous "needle test" that indicated we would have two girls! Two babies would be a beautiful challenge. I can't wait to see how things will unfold.

Not all journeys start the same way, at least not with a diagnosis. Mine begins with a lot of hope and good news. My exams are good, my partner's too, inseminations are covered by Health Insurance, and the clinic is extraordinary. Everything seemed to indicate that the word infertility was just a brief passage in our lives.

OCTOBER 4, 2021

That's it! I had the first ultrasound and started taking medication. I have 10 follicles on the right and 9 follicles on the left. Maybe you are somewhere in there! The medication I'm taking makes me very tired, and to my surprise, it is also used to treat breast cancer. Weird! The next ultrasound is on October 8, and we will have the date of the insemination then. I can't wait. Time is not moving fast enough for me, but we're slowly preparing for your arrival. We moved the guest room and painted everything. Your bedroom will have a touch of green.

I couldn't help but research every step, every medication. I wanted to know exactly what was happening in my body. So, as I still had my medication guide from my auxiliary nurse class, I religiously looked up all the information about Letrozole, as if it were an exam question. To my great surprise, what is now stimulating my ovaries to produce mature eggs was also used to treat breast cancer. I thought of a family friend, the great Lulu Hughes. She had fought breast cancer. I remember the time I had to give her a subcutaneous injection in her belly just before a show. As I recalled this memory, I suddenly felt very close to her. Our struggles were certainly not the same, but they were women's struggles, and if I could have a third of her courage, then I would make it.

OCTOBER 8, 2021

Today, I had my second ultrasound. I have good news and bad news. The good news is that I will trigger my ovulation tonight at 11pm, and the insemination is scheduled for October 10. My egg on the right is 20 mm, which seems to be a very good size, and I'm super excited. The bad news is that the doctor who did the ultrasound saw that my left fallopian tube is dilated and blocked. And that's not good! If I'm not pregnant 16 days after insemination, I'll have to undergo surgery. They'll have to see what's going on with that fallopian tube and if the problem can be fixed. They will also check if the right one is healthy. If the problem can't be resolved, I'll have to start thinking about in vitro fertilization. If I'm pregnant 16 days later, I'll be a "high-risk pregnancy," and I'll have to have an ultrasound at 6 weeks to make sure I'm not having an ectopic pregnancy, which could kill you and me too. I keep hoping that everything will be fine. That's what Stef and Yza, my father's girlfriend, tell me, but it's hard not to think about it! One thing at a time. Being worried and excited at the same time is very strange. It's like two feelings that don't go together at all, and the more excited I am, the more worried I am. Should I stop thinking about it? Impossible! I'm positive, but after news like that, how can I be 100% positive? I'll keep thinking about you, and everything should be fine. One thing is for sure, I want you, and it's hard to wait for you. We could say that I loved you before I even knew you.

A dilated and blocked fallopian tube is called hydrosalpinx! It's an infection that creates fluid in the fallopian tube, and no, you can't cure it with antibiotics. There is an operation to unblock the tube and remove the fluid, but it will inevitably come back. After bad news about our health, we tend to want to find a solution. We ask, "What are the treatments, Doctor?" In my case, what was peculiar was that we were going to try insemination before doing an operation on the tubes. I could have canceled the insemination and postponed it. But since my right tube was healthy, and my mature egg was on the right, there was a good chance that everything would go well. In short, we wait to see if the worst happens before treating the problem. I never thought that in addition to not being able to have a child naturally, we would be talking about possible complications and surgeries. All this scared me, but did I really have the right to complain? It was I, who wanted a child, and I was solely responsible for what happened to me. My hydrosalpinx was due to an untreated chlamydia. How could I have missed that? In doing research, I learned that chlamydia is asymptomatic about fifty percent of the time.

I've already had sex education classes, so why didn't I know that? I was too trustful and not rigorous enough with screening tests. I was very ashamed of myself, I felt humiliated to have to explain the cause of my problem. I was guilty of all my misfortunes, but if I wanted to move forward, I had to start accepting and above all, assuming that unprotected sex had irreversibly damaged an important part of my reproductive system. Quite a heavy punishment for such a short pleasure.

OCTOBER 10, 2021

That's it! It's done! You might be growing in my belly right now. I hope with all my heart! I don't know how I'm going to wait 16 days before taking a pregnancy test. I probably won't be able to. This is so exciting, I lack words. I already feel pregnant. It seems that all uncertainties have disappeared. There's only positivity, happiness, love, and excitement. I can't wait to take a test and know that you're right there with me, in my belly.

I had finally undergone the insemination. A quick and painless procedure that would allow me to have a child. I still remember the orange walls at the clinic. A few days earlier, Yza had told me that the color of the reproduction chakra was orange and that I should surround myself with this color as much as possible. The doctor informed me, "It's over! You can lie down for 5 minutes and leave afterward." In the end, I stayed for 15 minutes, with my hands on my lower abdomen, staring at the orange walls. I am extremely close to Yza. Several years ago, she went through this as well. She has polycystic ovary syndrome and has made several attempts to have a child. She told me her story only once, and to her surprise, it was the first time she told it all without crying. We have a very strong bond, and every time we're together, we experience very intense moments. Unfortunately, after losing her twins, she decided to stop. This summer, after I had sent her a photo of my blooming roses, and she replied:

"Oh wow! Do you know that I named my twin fetuses Rose and Blanche. It still moves me when I see a white rose! Thank you for this moment of tenderness in my heart. Your rose bushes are beautiful, my peanut." I love you so much, Yza.

OCTOBER 23, 2021

Finally! A positive test this morning and a second one tonight! I'm on cloud nine, my body is shaking! I am so happy; I feel like I've won the lottery! It's like a miracle. You're here, inside me, cozy and warm in my belly! Welcome home, my angel. I love you, and I will take care of you. Tomorrow I will take another test to make sure I'm not dreaming!

Do you remember the most beautiful Christmas gift you ever received as a child? Do you remember your reaction? The big smile from ear to ear? The screams? The tears? The feeling that it was the best day of your life, that nothing else mattered? Well, imagine that feeling amplified when my eyes met the two pink lines that announced life.

OCTOBER 24, 2021

Third POSITIVE test! I know you're here; I can feel you! I am overjoyed! Tomorrow, I will start the procedures, call the clinic and my employer.

OCTOBER 25, 2021

Today, I am officially on preventive leave, and tomorrow, I will have a blood test to confirm my pregnancy. I can't wait! I will focus on you and me. My little miracle, I can't wait to see you, touch you, feel you. Not just me, everyone is excited to see you.

It's the kind of news that's hard to keep to yourself. How to keep silent when I'm jumping up and down? Anyway, there's a light in my face that can't be hidden. The joy was so intense that not for a second was I afraid or in doubt. I had completely forgotten about this story of hydrosalpinx and surgery. I shouted from the rooftops that I was carrying life, blinded by the image of a sweet and perfect future.

OCTOBER 26, 2021

I had my blood test this morning, and I got my result. My pregnancy is confirmed, but my hormone levels are not as high as they should be. I'm at 81, and I should be above 100. It doesn't worry me; the nurse told me it could be due to the delay in my ovulation. According to the results chart, it would mean that I'm theoretically 4 weeks pregnant, but it doesn't matter! It doesn't matter! The important thing is that you are here and healthy. My whole family knows now, and on Friday, we will announce it to Stef's family. Tomorrow, I'll do another blood test to see if my hormones have doubled. I can't stop thinking about you all the time! I already love you so much; I hope you feel it.

Oh, I'm sure this little cell has felt a lot of love. Pure and unconditional love. Despite the warning that was the result of this blood test, my head told my heart that maybe if I sent enough love, everything would be fine! But when I received my second result, slowly, my little white cloud began its descent into hell.

OCTOBER 28, 2021

I had my second blood test, and the nurse wasn't pleased with the results. My hormones should have doubled. I was at 81 last time, and if I remember correctly, I'm now at 115. She made me understand that I'm theoretically 4.4 weeks pregnant, which makes no sense for the hormone level I'm at. I asked her honestly what that meant. She said either you're taking your time to grow and not growing fast, or I'm having a chemical pregnancy, which would mean I have an empty gestational sac: a house, no baby. It worries me a little. I don't know what to think. My joy has become so fragile, and I feel like at any moment I could hear bad news and lose you. I remain positive because it feels like you're there; maybe you're shy about showing yourself. The nurse wants me to have another blood test on November 1 to see how it evolves and eventually have my first ultrasound in six weeks to hear your little heart. I will cry so much when I hear your heart beating inside my belly. All I have to do now is take care of me and you, and wait for time to work its magic. The nurse told me to watch out for worrying symptoms, but for now, I have none, so it's encouraging. I don't know how Stef sees all this. It must be difficult for him to sort this all out; it's not happening in his belly, but your grandmother will pray for us, for you!

Of course, Stef is worried, but he doesn't know how to react. I see the light in his eyes when he announces to someone that I'm pregnant. However, you can hear the worry in his voice when he says that I'm having several blood tests and that we need to monitor certain symptoms. As it is still possible that everything will turn out fine, he keeps a lot inside to avoid scaring me.

NOVEMBER 2, 2021

I received the result of my third blood test this morning, and I am at 306. I should be above 400. We will stop the blood tests because we are clearly in a gray area. I will have my first ultrasound on November 8 to see if you are in the right place and another one a week later to see if your little heart is beating. In the meantime, I need to be attentive to symptoms of an ectopic pregnancy like heavy bleeding or severe pain in the lower abdomen. I must continue to take care of myself to maximize the chances of having a beautiful, healthy baby. I feel fine, but worried. I know you are there, but I don't know if you are okay. I'm afraid of having to say goodbye to you and having to start all over again. I want someone to tell me that everything is fine and that I will be able to hold you in my arms very soon.

As you may suspect, I never made it to that ultrasound appointment. It took me 4 days before I was able to write the following. It was as painful to live as it was to write. It still is today.

NOVEMBER 10, 2021

I'm sorry, my angel! I don't want to hurt you. I don't want to kill you; I don't want you to leave me. I have no choice but to end my pregnancy... I have an ectopic pregnancy. You're not in the right place, my angel, you can't survive where you are, and neither can I. It kills me to have to do this because you were on a good path. You were growing well, and I had to stop everything. I feel like I'm killing you intentionally, like I don't want you. If you only knew how much I wanted you in my life. I can't do anything, change anything, and now you are dying in my womb and you will disappear like bruises disappear after a while, when we bump into something. A pain that disappears but is never forgotten. It all started on November 6 at 1:30 p.m... Stef and I were at the market, and I had sharp pains in the lower right abdomen. We went to the emergency room, and I was quickly classified as priority 2. When I entered the doctor's office, I started bleeding. The doctor did a scan of my abdomen and ordered a blood test. There was blood accumulating in the abdomen. When we got the results, it was strange because my pregnancy hormones had increased. I was at 1800. Then the on-call gynecologist examined me to better understand what was happening to me and make a decision. It was 8 p.m., and she decided to keep me overnight with a saline solution, blood tests every 4 hours, and fasting from midnight. I spent the night in the emergency room corridor on a stretcher, and it was not easy. The next day, my hormones increased well, and so did my hemoglobin. I had an ultrasound, and they saw that I had ovarian cysts. My tubes were intact, but still no embryo in sight. So, the gynecologist let me go home with 24-hour surveillance. I had an appointment on November 9 at 9 a.m. at the high-risk pregnancy clinic at the hospital. They started by taking a blood test. The result was 4200 for my hormones. Very good evolution. Then I had an ultrasound because at this level of HCG, we can see the embryonic sac. There was nothing in my uterus. The only thing they could see was a hematoma next to my right ovary, which could be a ruptured cyst. That would explain my lower abdominal pain. Because the doctor couldn't see the embryonic sac in my uterus, she diagnosed an ectopic pregnancy. It destroyed me. I'm still destroyed, but I can't change anything, and it's very hard for me. Then I had two injections (like chemotherapy) to stop cell division. Sorry, I'm having a hard time. I love you...

I struggled to breathe, feeling as though my breath had been momentarily cut off. Tears streamed down my face, blurring my vision so severely that I couldn't even see what I was writing. After my trip to the hospital, I was gripped with fear, dreading the possibility of receiving bad news. Sitting at the high-risk pregnancy clinic among expectant mothers gently cradling their swollen bellies, I couldn't help but hope for the chance to experience that joy myself soon. Their obliviousness to my envy was understandable, but it weighed heavily on me. As the wait stretched on endlessly, Stef, who attempted to be present for the appointment, had to leave for the start of his shift. In my state of denial, I reassured him that everything would be fine and urged him to leave. Regret filled him later, evident in his face during our Facetime call after the diagnosis was delivered.

The hour I spent waiting for the pharmacy to supply methotrexate felt interminable. Unable to endure the company of expectant mothers any longer, I stepped outside. The pain I felt was already overwhelming; there was no need to compound it further. Navigating my way out of the hospital proved difficult, as grief clouded my senses, causing me to pause repeatedly to regain my composure and clear my tear-blurred vision. Passersby, concerned by my distress, offered inquiries about my well-being, to which I mechanically replied with a strained "I'm fine," though the truth was far from it.

Once outside, I called my mother, seeking her love and compassion. Seeing my distress, she came to join me. Overwhelmed by emotion, we sat on the grass in front of the hospital, finding comfort in each other's embrace. It was then that I received the call informing me that the methotrexate had arrived. The sight of those two syringes filled with fluorescent yellow liquid, to be handled with gloved hands, will forever be etched in my memory.

Ironically, with the high-risk pregnancy clinic closed, I was escorted to the maternity ward to receive my injections. In the very place where life is celebrated, I found myself losing yours. That day, something within me shattered irreparably.

NOVEMBER 12, 2021

Today, I had my second appointment at the high-risk pregnancy clinic. Not a great day. I received two more doses of methotrexate, and it's still as painful physically and emotionally. Especially since I could hear a heartbeat coming from the room next door. The nurse called me later to give me the results of my HCG. I am at 6342... It continues to increase, and at the next appointment, I will have to wait for the result before getting another dose or seeing the gynecologist again. I'm not exactly sure what will happen, but I hope I won't have to undergo surgery. It really scares me! It's been a tough day... I still struggle to understand how I'm going to get through this.

Once again, I found myself sitting in that waiting room surrounded by pregnant women. There was this girl sitting across from me, talking on the phone. She was telling the person on the other end that she already had 3 children and didn't want any more. She had come to make sure everything was okay for her abortion.

Did she know what I was going through? No!

Could she have been more discreet about the reason for her presence? Most definitely!

Did I, deep inside, want to throw a chair in her face? Absolutely!

Somewhere between grief and rage, I promised myself that if I ever got pregnant, I would maintain discretion and restraint in public. You never know what the girl next to you is going through. Stef was holding my hand, and I could see the pain and sorrow in his eyes. There was nothing he could do to ease the heaviness pressing on my chest, a weight that was making it hard for me to breathe with each injection. Every time the nurse injected a dose, it felt like my throat was being seared with a hot iron. I was in tears, and Stef could only keep me from crashing down, as we exited the hospital.

NOVEMBER 15, 2021

Once again today, I had a blood test, and I'm not expecting good news because my breasts are sore. As expected, my hormone levels have risen above 9000, so the methotrexate isn't working. I'll have to undergo surgery today. The gynecologist explained everything to me, and she will likely remove my left fallopian tube, as it is damaged and that's where you are. You have no chance of surviving where you are, and I'm sorry because I have no way out either, no hope of a miracle. It's over, and they are preparing me for the surgery. I'm terrified. As I enter the day surgery clinic, Stef is getting ready to go to work. My father is on his way to join me. At 5:20 pm, I went in for the operation. I met the gynecologist, the nurse, and the anesthesiologist, and then I entered the operating room. I couldn't help but cry; I was scared. They prepared me, gave me oxygen, and suddenly, I was gone! When I woke up, the first thing I felt was pain, both physical and psychological. My body was trembling, the gas in my body was compressing my lungs, and yet, I felt empty. It took me 40 minutes to wake up, and the more I regained consciousness, the more I wished I could continue sleeping. The gynecologist who operated on me had returned to the maternity ward, so all they could tell me about the operation was that they had removed a fallopian tube.

I felt empty, both physically and mentally consumed by pain. It was probably the closest I've been to experience depression. My body refused to cooperate, I couldn't even sit up without assistance, relying on support to move around. Thankfully, my father stepped in to care for me while Stef was at work. Never being alone probably saved me from spiraling further.

Ariel, a compassionate coworker, also extended her helping hand while awaiting my father's arrival. She humorously noted the parallels between my requests and our work duties as she assisted me in getting up, walking to the bathroom, and even heating up my meals. Despite the agony I was in, her infectious smile and playful demeanor never failed to bring a moment of levity. With her encouragement, 'Alright, Mrs. Plante, lean on me, let's get moving! Off to the bathroom we go. Need help with your pants?' I couldn't help but crack a smile, despite the pain. That evening, she provided me with the support I needed most. Thank you, Ariel!"

NOVEMBER 18, 2021

Today, the gynecologist who operated on me called. In the end, the operation didn't go as we had imagined. The ectopic pregnancy was on the right side and had severely damaged my fallopian tube. So, it's the right tube that she removed. That was my healthy tube! The left tube is also damaged by hydrosalpinx, but she couldn't make the decision to sterilize me during the operation without my consent. We are still disappointed, and the stream of bad news shows no signs of stopping. I called my fertility clinic. The receptionist told me not to cancel my appointments, that the doctors at the clinic would review my hospital file and discuss the best options with me. The doctor from the emergency room also reached out to me, inquiring about my well-being. I shared my current state of mind, and as we wrapped up the call, she expressed her willingness to monitor any future pregnancies. I found that deeply moving; it felt like a soothing balm to my heart, given the ongoing challenges. I can't wait for my body to return to its normal state. I long for my heart to heal.

It was at that moment that I understood. Even though no one dared to say it that way, I was sterile. The world had just come crashing down on me... 25 years old and sterile... Everyone else's problems seemed so small and insignificant. It's important to mention that all of this unfolds during the COVID-19 pandemic. Everyone was complaining about trivial issues, and my frustration with the world was only just beginning.

NOVEMBER 30, 2021

This morning, I received a call from a doctor who could perform surgery. An operation to assess the condition of my fallopian tube. She gave me 4 options.

1. *No operation and we try insemination.*
2. *No operation and we try in vitro fertilization.*

3. *Operation to try to repair my tube.*
4. *Operation to remove the fallopian tube (salpingectomy).*

I feel at loss and I'm not sure what to do. I feel like my best option is the worst option. I looked online, and everything seems to suggest that I should have a salpingectomy. I'm the only one who can make this decision, and I feel like I'm alone in the world, and no one can help me. I don't know if I'll be able to get through the holidays if I go back to work. I would need someone to talk to about all this, someone who wants to be there for me. Stef is here, but he doesn't know how to handle all this, and I would need someone neutral. I feel like that person will never come, and I'll have to face all this alone in my head.

We had never been so emotionally distant from each other. While he needed me and I needed him, bridging the gap seemed impossible. I had just experienced the toughest moment of my life, and on his end, his friendships were beginning to falter. No more calls, texts or visits—it even felt awkward to invite us to social events. He felt isolated and found it deeply unsettling to be excluded because we had chosen to start a family. People assumed I was pressuring him into parenthood. What frustrated us both, was that everyone had their own opinion on the matter, but no one bothered to ask about our plans nor offered any support. They all cited his best friend, who couldn't grasp why we were pursuing this path. He would tell us, "If it's not happening naturally, why force it? Spending so much money on it seems absurd." When I began talking about in vitro fertilization, and its associated costs, suddenly, our project seemed ridiculous. It was easy for him to pass judgement, he had four children. Easy for him to criticize when he hadn't faced the challenges we were faced with. Secretly, I resented him for not understanding. It seemed as though he was determined to change Stef's mind. I found myself alone in defending our choices, struggling to uphold my own spirits, and supporting Stef as best I could. Let's not forget, he too had just lost a child.

JANUARY 20, 2022

It's been a while since I last wrote in my journal. I guess I was too caught up with my emotions to take a moment and write them down. There have been countless tears and countless nights filled with anguish. While I have been fortunate enough to be part of a support group, your absence continues to weigh heavily on my heart, leaving a wound that I fear will never heal completely. Am I a mother? I think so. My heart has changed, I can feel it. I now have an angel somewhere who, I hope, is watching over me. I received a call from a doctor at my fertility clinic offering a bit of hope through a different approach. Despite the challenges posed by my condition, she mentioned the possibility of success if certain factors align. I'm scheduled for tests during the next cycle, and we'll take it from there. Every day is a battle to keep my spirits up. Returning to work has been particularly challenging, as I can't help but imagine how far along I would have been by now. Despite the sadness, I cling to the hope that one day soon, I'll have the joy of holding you in my arms. You are the missing piece that completes my life.

After the surgery, I was relieved to be presented with a plan that didn't require further operations. Recovering physically had been tough enough, and all I wanted now, was to nurture my mental well-being. I was deeply convinced that I had to spare no effort in order to get better. Work was however very challenging. I kept wondering how I could possibly provide optimal care to my patients, while feeling in desperate need of support myself. Amidst this emotional turmoil, there was Mrs Rita, a remarkable 101-year-old lady. I had been assigned to her care, which involved providing for her well-being and guiding the staff in making decisions for her. She had slowly become my motivation to go to work, as we grew closer to one another and developed a trusting bond. In moments of clarity, I confided in her about my infertility journey, and she listened attentively. Though I suspected she might not grasp every detail, she never failed to express gratitude at the end of our conversations, unaware of the profound impact she had on me.

JANUARY 22, 2022

We are not eligible for the free public program for assisted reproduction. So, we will have to pay for all treatments from now on. I want you with all my heart, and I will fight for you. I have set up a GoFundMe to raise money for the treatments. I feel so bad asking people for money, but I won't be able to do it alone. I feel bad, and with every donation, I burst into tears. I just hope that in the end, the treatments work, and I can have my family. My child. My miracle.

It took every ounce of courage to set up this GoFundMe. With each donation we received, waves of guilt washed over me, often accompanied by tears. Witnessing the kindness and generosity of strangers towards our cause was deeply moving. Yet, there was a part of me that couldn't shake the feeling of shame when addressing the issue of hydrosalpinx. With a bit of research, people would understand my condition. However, I refused to give up! I was saving money like never before, and the GoFundMe would give me a much-needed boost.

JANUARY 26, 2022

With my savings and my GoFundMe campaign, we have already raised $2,500. It's a start! I received my ovulation and pregnancy tests, so the only thing left is to do the hysterosalpingography to get the ball rolling. I'm really excited because it will be the decisive *moment for me, to see if I have a chance of getting pregnant without in vitro fertilization.*

One morning, I was taken aback by a message on Facebook from a friend. It read, 'If you give me a dollar, I'll give you a dollar,' along with a GoFundMe link. He was soliciting donations to buy a video game, citing it as his long-held dream. He even went to the extent of making a video, but I never got the courage to watch it. I couldn't help but interpret it as a mockery of my own fundraising campaign. It felt like he was trivializing my struggles. His lack of consideration left me feeling deeply hurt and resentful, especially given all that I had endured. Despite my friend's usual sensitivity towards mental health issues, he seemed oblivious to the impact of his actions on my emotional well-being. To this day, I struggle to comprehend how some individuals can be so tactless when interacting with those facing fertility challenges. It's a painful reminder that our experiences are often underestimated and misunderstood."

FEBRUARY 11, 2022

Today, my appointment at the fertility clinic didn't go quite as I imagined. I was supposed to have an ovarian ultrasound and a hysterosalpingography, to assess the condition of my fallopian tube. The doctor performed the ultrasound, and everything seemed alright. There was no need for the hysterosalpingography because, just from the ultrasound, he could see that my tube was blocked and highly infected. Insemination would be pointless, so we're moving directly to in vitro fertilization. For the fresh embryo transfer, I will keep my fallopian tube. Should the transfer fail though, I will have to have it removed and do a frozen embryo transfer afterward. I'm already on the waiting list, and it should bring us to this summer. I'm already looking forward to starting and doing something concrete to have my miracle. It's been a while since I've only been living with uncertainties, and I can't wait to see positive results. The doctor is preparing my protocol, and I have an appointment soon to confirm the in vitro fertilization.

MARCH 10, 2022

Big news today: I received an email from my fertility clinic informing me that I can start my in vitro fertilization protocol on April 12th. I'm so happy to be able to start earlier than expected; it's completely surreal! With the GoFundMe campaign and our savings, we've raised $5,000. I know I shouldn't get ahead of myself because even though the fallopian tube complication is ruled out, there may be other bumps along the way. Nevertheless, I'm hopeful that everything will go well, and we'll have our little miracle soon.

APRIL 7, 2022

Today is a special day because I finally have raised enough money to pay for all my treatments. I'm ready to start the medication and get a little closer to you.

APRIL 20, 2022

Finally, my day 1! I'm starting the medication, and I'm super excited! I can't wait to see the progress of my follicles on the ultrasounds. I hope everything goes well.

Every evening, during my dinner break and at the end of the shift, Stef would come join me at the nursing station to administer my injections. It didn't hurt at all. All our colleagues showed interest in this peculiar process. Sometimes, the nurses would glance at us to see if we were mastering the techniques. I would prepare the syringes, and Stef would administer the injections. Since I completed all my practical and theoretical training as a licensed practical nurse, I had a very good understanding of injections, and I was proud of it.

MAY 2, 2022

It's been 9 days since I started the injections, and thankfully, still no symptoms of hyperstimulation or side effects from the medications. Stef has perfected his injection technique and has almost become a pro at it. Today, I had my third ultrasound, and everything looks good. Tomorrow is my last day of stimulation, and then we trigger my ovulation. The egg retrieval is coming!

MAY 4, 2022

I stimulated my ovulation with two injections. Tomorrow, I have a day off from injections; I'll only need to take antibiotics. On May 6th, it's the day of the egg retrieval. I'm somewhat stressed out about the pain I might feel, but overall, I'm really excited for the experience! Each day, I remind myself that my body is working hard and that I'm privileged to have access to this kind of treatment. I eagerly anticipated every injection, and now that I've had them all, I'm confident that the rewards of these efforts will soon be realized.

MAY 6, 2022

This morning, I arrived at the clinic at 8 a.m. for my egg retrieval procedure. I put on my cap and small hospital gown, and then the nurse inserted an intravenous catheter. She was really friendly, and I was quite nervous. Once in the operating room however, I felt very calm. They even asked me what music I wanted to listen to. You came out of my body for the first time to The Beatles. I hardly felt any pain, and I was completely captivated by the screen where I could see each of my follicles being retrieved. They retrieved 15 eggs from me, and I witnessed each one of them carefully leaving my body. I found it beautiful. I found it more than beautiful; it was magnificent! Each little egg was potentially a baby that would grow inside me. The nurse was singing beside me, and there was a cheerful atmosphere in the operating room. It was a very beautiful moment filled with gentleness and joy.

MAY 7, 2022

Yesterday, an hour after the retrieval, we received a call from the lab. On my side, everything is fine; I have 15 mature eggs. Unfortunately, the sperm isn't moving. They don't want to risk fertilizing my eggs with dead sperm. My eggs will be frozen, and we won't be able to do a fresh transfer. At least not until we have good sperm. We're disappointed because we were sure that this time would be the right one.

Every time we encounter another obstacle or waiting period, it's a profound disappointment. We were so sure of ourselves, believing it would be a smooth journey to pregnancy, and we faced yet another setback. For Stef, it was really disconcerting because suddenly, he was the one with a problem. Despite my attempts to reassure him that every challenge has a solution, he couldn't shake off the growing sense of discouragement. On the phone, with a lot of empathy, the nurse asked us to come back in two days to provide another sample. While we hoped for a positive outcome, deep down, we understood that it wouldn't be that simple. We braced ourselves for the possibility of receiving unfavorable news.

MAY 9, 2022

Stef gave 2 samples today, and the news wasn't good. There is no sperm in his semen. I'm completely devastated! Why is it so hard for us? As soon as one thing goes well, something else ruins it all! When it's not me who's not functioning, it's him. My doctor suggested something to us, and we accepted. Stef will undergo surgery. A urologist will retrieve sperm directly from his testicles. It's the simplest and quickest method. We have to wait for the call to schedule an appointment. That's the only thing that deeply annoys me... We don't know when it will happen.

MAY 11, 2022

Plot twist! This morning, we received a call from my fertility clinic saying the urologist was on-site and available not only to meet Stef but also to perform the surgery today! A stroke of luck in our misfortune. It felt good to have a little boost of hope. Stef was a bit stressed, but overall, it went really well. $2,500 later, aside from some pain for Stef, we had 15 samples of beautiful, mobile sperm, which is excellent news. Everything was frozen, and now we wait for the next step.

Now that we had all our samples frozen, we were really looking forward to the call from the clinic, knowing that we were just one step away from a possible pregnancy. We were already arranging the house and the yard for a growing family. Our impatience returned, but this time, it was filled with positivity. We found ourselves dreaming of the changes and joys that our baby would bring into our lives.

MAY 17, 2022

Today, I received a call from the IVF coordinator, and she wanted to know my next day 1. It's perfect timing because it's today! She said it would be safer to wait another cycle because my eggs will probably be large, and I might develop post-retrieval cysts. I really don't want to wait another cycle, so I made an appointment for an ultrasound on May 19th. This ultrasound will tell us if everything is okay or not. I still trust my body because I feel great, as if I had never had all those injections and the retrieval. I'm ready!

As I was about to embark on the final step toward pregnancy, I lost my confidante at work, that centenarian lady who had helped me find my motivation at work, who had made me laugh, and who had listened to me so well during my difficult moments. Dear Mrs. Rita has passed away. We had already begun her palliative care a while ago, and our conversations had turned into moments of relaxation. With soft piano and violin music playing. When I entered her room, I hardly needed to speak anymore because she knew the gentleness of my care. One day, at the beginning of my shift, her son informed me that the medication had not relieved her discomfort all day. When I finished giving her care, she finally seemed relieved and serene. A few minutes later, her son called me out into the hallway to tell me she had passed away. In my mind, I'm convinced she waited for me. Perhaps to say thank you or goodbye? Or to tell me that everything would be okay. I felt such great sadness. She was so luminous. I would have loved to have known her before her illness. This great lady was a pillar in the most difficult moment of my life, and I will never forget her. Thank you, Mrs. Rita.

MAY 19, 2022

I had my ultrasound, and even though my ovaries are enlarged and I have residues of hemorrhagic cysts, my doctor gave me the green light to start the medication. I'm really pleased to be able to start now. I feel truly ready to undergo the transfer. I can't wait for it to become a reality and not just a dream. So, medication from day 3 to day 7, and then another ultrasound on May 25th. I hope this is it!

MAY 25, 2022

I had my ultrasound, and we'll have to wait a bit. My largest follicle is at 13 mm, and my doctor said we want to reach at least 18 mm. So, we scheduled another appointment for May 28th, and in the meantime, I have to do ovulation tests to make sure I don't miss it. It's really hard to always be in a state of waiting, but I think it will make the experience even more extraordinary. I'm dreading

July a bit. It's the month when, normally, I should have been giving birth. It feels strange to think that I should have a big belly right now. My angel is in heaven, and I eagerly await my little miracle.

MAY 28, 2022

I just got back from my ultrasound appointment, and I'm overjoyed! It's getting serious now. She gave me the OK to continue, so tomorrow, I'll trigger my ovulation. On May 31st, they will thaw my eggs and the sperm, and they'll perform fertilization. On June 5th, I'll have my transfer, and on June 16th, my blood test. Imagine that, 10 days before my birthday, a beautiful positive result. It would be such a wonderful gift. If only time could pass quickly until then!

We were finally at the finish line of this long marathon, and nothing could cloud my joy. It was finally the long-awaited moment. Stef remained cautious because we had been so hurt when we lost the baby. He said he would truly be happy when I have a big belly, and even though I understood the fear that gripped him. On my end, I couldn't contain my excitement.

JUNE 1, 2022

15 eggs warmed, 14 eggs micro-injected, 12 eggs fertilized. That's the tally for the day! Out of 15, 12 have survived and are now developing. We'll receive more news about our little ones on June 3rd. In the meantime, I'm taking my progesterone to prepare my body to welcome a miracle.

JUNE 3, 2022

Today, the embryologist called me and said I had 9 high-quality embryos. He confirmed that my transfer will indeed be on Sunday. I can't wait to see my perfect little cell.

JUNE 5, 2022

This morning, the embryologist called me before my appointment to tell me I had a 5AA embryo, which is the best quality. The others will be kept under observation until tomorrow to see how they evolve, and then they'll be frozen. I finally had my transfer. At 10 a.m., I saw my little miracle, a small white ball, gently settling into my uterus, holding Stef's hand. A wonderful feeling. As if, this time, it was the real deal. I hope you'll hold on.

It was the most beautiful thing in the world to see that little white ball gently settle into my uterine lining. After the transfer, the nurse and doctor congratulated us with their biggest smiles, and once in the car, my hand on my belly, I felt light and lucky. The fertility journey is not something fun, but I thought I was lucky to see my little embryo, barely a few millimeters, descend into my uterus. At that moment, there was no word strong enough to describe what I felt. All that was left was to wait for confirmation of this miracle.

JUNE 16, 2022

Today, I went for my blood test at the clinic, and I'm awaiting the results in the early afternoon. I'm quite positive because I took three pregnancy tests, and they were all positive. I'm really looking forward to receiving this call... I'm super happy! My levels are at 736. That's seven times higher than my first pregnancy. It's the real deal! I'll have my first ultrasound on July 4th, and I'm really excited to see you where you belong.

I was so happy with all these good news! However, we kept our composure knowing that I had a damaged fallopian tube due to hydrosalpinx and that the embryo could travel up to it. There was still a small risk of ectopic pregnancy, but when I received the results of my blood test, I felt that this time, it was for real.

JULY 4, 2022

We went for the ultrasound, and it was magical. Right from the first image, the baby is in the right place. The second thing I noticed was its little heart! I didn't hear it, but I saw it moving. It was wonderful! I'm on cloud nine, with a beautiful 9.3 mm baby filling me with immense happiness.

I never wrote in this journal again; those were my last words. I could finally close this chapter of my life. I can't describe the feeling I had when I saw those images; it was an intense sense of victory and pride. It was as if I had lifted the weight of the world off my shoulders. Tears filled our eyes. I never thought I would experience all of this. I went through a range of emotions, sometimes feeling several at once. Today, I know that it was all completely normal.

I will never forget the loss of my baby. That wound will never fully heal. I'm proud of my journey, but to this day, there's a part of me that still feels ashamed. A guilt for putting myself through all of this because of past mistakes. Maybe one day I'll be able to accept it, but I feel like it will be a lifelong journey. I found beauty through my journey, which probably helped me find the procedures less painful. I found answers when I had questions, thanks to the online support group. I found inspiring people to give me strength in my moments of weakness, thank you to Yza and Lulu. I found people to make me laugh when I felt like crying, thank you Ariel. I found help when I thought I was alone, thank you to all my generous donors. I found people to listen to me when my heart was heavy, thank you Mrs Rita. I found a shoulder to cry on when I needed it, thank you mom. I found someone to take care of me in my moments of solitude, thank you dad. I found a hand to hold when I was in pain, thank you my love. I found someone to encourage me, thank you to my best friend.

To all the women experiencing infertility, I say this: Find what brings you comfort, what helps you, find the beauty hidden in your journey. You work hard and you deserve gentleness.

Today, with humility, I share with you the first few lines of the beginning of a new journal.

FEBRUARY 24, 2023

I'm struggling to grasp what just happened. It's been 27 hours since I last slept, 12 hours that the contractions have been driving me crazy, and 2 hours of pushing with all my might. It's 2:11 PM, and the doctor has just placed you on me. At that precise moment, I met Romy, and she is undoubtedly the most beautiful thing I've ever seen in my life.

I have finally found my miracle.

CHAPTER 4

A PREGNANCY AT WHAT COST?

By Virginie Bisson

The migraines were intense. You know, the kind of pain that makes you want to smash your head against the wall or struggle to simply open your eyes. I had to do something, it just didn't make any sense to keep going with this much pain and pressure in the upper face. This grand decision which was going to literally turn my life upside down was therefore taken one evening of October 2018, right there in my kitchen, with the lights dimmed down in an effort to conjure the pain.

— "I think I'm going to stop taking the pill, my Love! I have read on the internet that migraines could be a side effect and, since we would like a child soon, why not? That would allow my body to get ready."

If we only had known at the time what was in store for us!

Two human beings in love, together for four years, wanting to start a family. It's simple, right?

So let me introduce myself. My name is Virginie Bisson. A small, feisty woman, standing at 5 feet tall, with brown hair, green eyes, and, most of all, a hard-headed nature, who refuses to back down or give up.

Life taught me that when you really want something, nothing is impossible! Surely, there are some exceptions, but God knows how much I want, how much I fought and am still fighting for this baby project. How much I overcame some of my most extreme fears and how much I still believe, to this day, that my turn will come. I sometimes wonder if I didn't create bad karma for myself.

You see, as a teenager, I kept telling my friends: "I will have kids at 21, but I'm worried about having infertility issues". Why did I say that? I've said it so many times! I'm not sure if one day I'll understand what was going through my head at the time. No one around me, back then, had any fertility issues. I had never even heard anything about it, whether on TV or on social media. Where did this fear come from? And I can hear people telling me: "Ah, that IS your problem! You think about it too much, that's why!"

I'll stop you right there. My story did not begin with the stress of procreation, and most of all, this sentence does not depict the situation: I was 23 at the time, freshly graduated as a professional kitchen designer. Jean-Simon, my Love, AKA J.S., had been an electrician for several years already and was 29. We were happily living on a campsite, year-round, in the hopes to save up and afford our own home and be able to welcome our newborn sooner than later.

— "What if we built it? There is no house to my liking and, between you and I, it's obvious we're in for endless renovations. Moreover, we all know it's not a good idea to mix renovations and a newborn. Also, that way, we'll be paying for something we really want! Oh, please say yes, my Love! I'll take care of everything, I promise!".

In that moment, I saw the most beautiful smile enlighten his face. One that meant all and everything. He was going to follow me in this inspiring project. Since we both work in the construction area, JS was not that difficult to convince in all honesty. Mind you, I've always known how to go about or find the right words to get me where I wanted to be (ok, I'm boasting a bit here!), but I must admit, the baby project managed to ground me and teach me to be patient.

After a few meetings with construction entrepreneurs, we were ready to begin this project. I had to unleash my creativity, but also, to try and have fun and feel stress free, with all that was happening. Everyone agreed that the best way to become pregnant was not to think about it. Nothing like building your own home to free your mind of a future pregnancy. And it was definitely the perfect occupation for me.

— "I just got the greatest idea, my Love! If I get pregnant soon, I'm going to give the contractor a choice of two colours and an envelope mentioning the sex of the baby, and then, he can paint the walls in the colour we picked for a boy or a girl. That way, we'll find out together, with our families, what's hidden in my belly."

We smiled at each other; we were so excited!

Construction was progressing well. Our minds were busy but each month that passed without a positive test weighed on our thoughts.

It was about a year later, after inconclusive attempts, and with a lump in my stomach, that I ended up asking my family doctor:

— "What if I had a problem?"

The doctor, always so self confident:

— "Give it time, Virginie! It will work soon, you're young. Still, I'm going to write you a referral for a fertility clinic, when you feel ready for it."

Entering the world of infertility means feeling alone amongst others. So many possible scenarios. Where to begin? Where to call? What questions to ask? It is not realizing right away how many women are going through this, when you feel so alone with your doctor's note, trying to get an appointment in a fertility clinic, trying to get help to understand your problem, but above all, to finally have a chance to realize your greatest wish, that of bearing life.

Talking openly about infertility, even to those close to you, can be so taboo and difficult, even today. Too many women live in silence with this stress, this suffering of the unknown.

And what to say about those close to you, uncomfortable around you, as if you were terminally ill, who almost avoid you, who don't dare saying anything for fear of not saying the right words, or even those who clumsily pass a comment, borderline inappropriate. But is there truly any right word?

For my part, I had the chance to meet a new friend, who happened to be part of this crazy journey as well. We were in the same high school, but not in the same circles, so we barely spoke to one another back then. Still, we were Facebook friends, at a time when it was the norm to add to your friends list any person you knew, even from afar. It was years after high school ended that we got closer, messaging each other after a post on indoor gardening I had published and that had captured her attention. During these exchanges, we realized we had so much in common, and were passionate about the same things. It was only a few weeks later that the subject of infertility was brought up and we realized we also had that in common. I mentioned I was lucky we were on the same boat but, between you and me, I would not even wish this on my worst enemy. I felt a bit selfish thinking I was not going to be alone, since I now had Sarah, the woman who would change my life and would be by my side on that hell of a roller coaster.

— "I'm scared, my friend. I'm afraid of needles, afraid of taking hormones and of the side effects they will have on my body. I'm scared of inseminations, but also terrified to lose control over my life. In my mind, it is totally unacceptable not to conceive naturally. I want to succeed alone and "normally". Why does everything have to be so complicated?'

— "I hear you, but isn't it about time to get the help you need and achieve your goal faster?"

Sarah always knew the right words, but also had that inner strength about her. She rushed head first and gave it all the courage she had to succeed in having her own miracle. Since she had applied for registration in a fertility clinic, I had to find the courage to dive in head first and get help as well.

I should tell you that just a few months prior, I would keep saying that it was out of the question for me to take hormones, to get inseminated and even more so to find myself in an IVF process. It seemed life had decided otherwise.

Both of us were going to have a baby and get to share that experience together. A tale of two best friends who get pregnant at the same time. Everyone's dream, right? This was the motivation I needed to take the first step. It took dozens of calls to finally have the right to my place in a clinic. Today, with the hindsight, I would have loved to have been better informed at that time, to have had someone to tell me to do research on multiple clinics in order to be better informed, instead of just choosing a clinic based on its location close to my home. But hey, in the end, every challenge in life teaches us something, whether it's a little or a lot, right?

— "Finally! I have my appointment to meet a fertility specialist, we're going to have our baby, my Love! Everything is going to be fine, I'm sure. Nothing can stop us! I hope...

I will always remember how stressed I was before my first appointment! What tests would I need to take? A camera in the crotch? Blood tests? A biopsy? Urine tests? What else? NOTHING? How do you mean, nothing? I was waiting in the gynecologist's office with only a pre-filled prescription for letrozole, he only had to sign it. Two or three formal questions. Thank you, next!

Still, I left the office with my motivation up high and yet another piece of paper. All I had to do was to wait for the famous day 1 of my next cycle and start taking the hormones. That seemed very simple. Letrozole on days 2 to 6 of the cycle, call the clinic when a home ovulation test was positive and, voilà! Insemination would be scheduled the next day. No ultrasound was planned during the cycle, no insemination on weekends was possible, so we crossed our fingers that I would ovulate during the week and ultimately no follow-up was done. It all seemed like a fit solution to get pregnant, right?

One, two and finally six insemination rounds ended up taking place in this same tiny room, white and cold, with the neon lights on the ceiling, where I was to find myself, the day after my ovulation, with my sperm sample tucked in my bra to keep it warm.

My spouse could not be present due to COVID-19. I kept telling myself that I was one of those women, ultra sensitive in the private area, or maybe I was just too stressed and scared and therefore probably more contracted, but each of these inseminations was painful for me, both physically and mentally. The thought of having to live through this hell again and again was unbearable. However, I couldn't bring myself to stop the process. I had already tried too hard. And this is how the mental exhaustion began creeping in on me. For some, this protocol would have been the perfect scenario for a future pregnancy. For me, it was simply... a waste of time? A hint of the world of infertility? I needed to understand or rather to have a truly professional medical care to feel confident. Am I wrong or every woman going through a journey in assisted reproduction has already said to herself: "Why is this so complicated when some women become pregnant simply by seeing a male organ?" My head was filled with questions.

— "Why can't I get pregnant? I am taking the medication as prescribed and, on top of that, I'm on my sixth insemination!"

It is suggested that I move on to the next step: in vitro fertilization. However, this means that I have to find a new clinic, because the one I go to does not offer this service. So, I end up waiting again for a spot in the health system... At the time, the idea of changing clinics discouraged me the most. Today I know it's the best thing that happened to me during this journey.

There has got to be several ways and solutions to try and feel good mentally, while experiencing this type of journey. Mine? Write up front on my Facebook page to talk about my infertility. I needed to scream to the whole world the evil that was inside me while making people aware of the subject. I also needed people to stop asking me: "Sooooo!" When is the baby due?" And then, I have to answer them very uncomfortably, a lump in the throat and a fake smile: "Ah! We will work on this soon."

It will have been a long personal journey, but also a mourning process to overcome. Because I dreamed more than anything of announcing a surprise pregnancy to my loved ones. The months passed one after another and so did my posts on social media and many women contacted me privately to talk about their own journey. To me, this was the best way to accept my condition, my new reality. Was this the right solution? Or rather, is there really a good solution? I couldn't say. To this day, there are unfortunately no books on how to cope with infertility. I knew deep down that I needed help, but I also wanted to help in my own way in return.

After a difficult depression caused by a false positive test that had created far too much joy, followed by unbearable suffering, what I needed most was to laugh. But first, let me take you back to this small trauma in my journey. That infamous November

9th, 2020. The day when, at last, I could see that second line on my pregnancy test. I had never had this chance before. I could clearly see that hoped-for line, and so could Jean-Simon. I must emphasize that, being a designer by trade, I work with colors. So, I have this unfortunate ability to see variations of white, even when just faint lines. If you knew the number of tests I did, when this second line was visible to my eyes, all the while JS would see the shadow of an "absolutely nothing ". But this time, it was really there! I took the test before dinner, because I had an incredible feeling. We couldn't even eat that evening because our bodies were overflowing with joy. I wanted to shout it from the rooftops, "FINALLY" and "Thank you, life." I had to show this test to someone else to confirm that I wasn't crazy. I immediately called my sister, who is a nurse, to come see it in person. She hugged me tightly and was so happy for us. The next day, she came to visit me at work to bring me two new pregnancy tests to take. Our family story, or rather our family journey, could finally begin. Unfortunately, the joy was very short-lived since the test the next day was negative, and so was the blood test. I will never really know what happened, but I know one thing: the pregnancy didn't progress. The call from my doctor to announce this negative result triggered my first major depression over my fertility issues. Unfortunately, it wouldn't be the last one in my journey, but I have always managed to pick myself up again. In the midst of all this, what I desperately needed was some kind of beauty in my life. It eventually turned into humorous videos on my TikTok account. I couldn't just live on the dark side of infertility, and I knew it. It wasn't always easy, clearly, but I had to be stronger. My journey has been a roller coaster from day one, but I do my best to stay as positive as possible. As I left the clinic after a routine ultrasound, my TikTok account skyrocketed with a viral video, giving me a total of over 10,000 followers and 1.7

million views to date. I have always been very shy and quite an introvert. I was able to add humor to my infertility journey on my platform. This brings me such an immense joy, more than I could ever fathom.

Many of us could recognize ourselves through these videos, and I knew it could make the process smoother for all these women, but especially for me. I feel less alone in this crazy journey. Honestly, who hasn't taken multiple pregnancy tests in the same day? Who hasn't tested at dpo8? Who has never taken a test when their periods were starting slowly? We are beautiful compulsive testers, let's stop hiding and share our reality.

So, it was time again to get back on a waiting list in hope for a spot in a private clinic. At that moment, luck was on my side. A new fertility clinic was about to open in my neighbourhood. The waiting time was shorter than waiting for a spot in other already established clinics. I got through right away during a first call one weekday evening in the parking lot of the grocery store. It was quite fast because, after sending the requested papers during the phone call, the registration was already completed with a spot in the clinic. So, a new chapter was beginning. I would finally be entitled to proper monitoring. Since no tests had been done before, it was time to catch up for real with endless blood tests, a hysteroscopy, a hysterosalpingography, and not to forget an endometrial biopsy. All this without counting the tests that my partner would have to undergo as well. After a few months of tests and waiting what seemed endless to me, we were finally ready to start a round of in vitro fertilization, following our classification as an unexplained infertility category. I was filled with mixed feelings between FINALLY and WHY ME? Receiving my prescription of a consequent amount of injection boxes and oral tablets generated intense stress and made me realize that we were actually starting this big step. It was time to buy a pill organizer to better manage each upcoming day.

It was a significant departure from the simple inseminations I had undergone previously, which lacked thorough medical monitoring. The process involved numerous new steps and procedures. I had been waiting for this moment so much, and I was so afraid. One weekday evening, sitting on my couch, I literally cried all the tears of my body imagining the upcoming steps that were finally coming too quickly.

I have a fear of needles. How will I manage to inject myself in the belly? It's impossible! Why do I have to go through this? Life is so unfair at times, I find.

"Shall we switch places, my love?"

"No, thank you! But please, know that I think you're extremely brave, really."

Jean-Simon is my best mental support, but we both know that if we were to actually switch places, this process would have been over a long time ago. He even repeated it to me several times laughing because JS's anxiety tends to want to take full control over his body. It would be too much to handle for him, and I respect that 100%. Fortunately for me, despite our fertility issues and our varied experiences with different clinics over the past three years, Sarah began her in vitro fertilization process just ten days before me.

What were the odds? However, it was perfect for taking the time to assimilate what was happening, and what better than a best friend to serve as a guinea pig for my first injection? Thank you, Sarah's belly! For her part, Sarah showed no stress and had absolute confidence in me. I found her brave for showing no weakness when she saw me with the injection pen in my hands, about to poke her, shaking like a leaf and I with absolutely no confidence in myself. In another life, I would never have agreed to do this. My turn would come very soon, and I had to be brave.

I didn't have a choice, and I knew it. Postponing the moment wouldn't help. A deep breath, and we insert. For my part, there was also a trembling of the hands from top to bottom and from left to right, all while pressing that damn pen plunger. The photo taken by my partner at that moment was prettier than the technique itself, but I would have many other moments to practice on myself. However, it was the biggest stress in the universe that was slowly diminishing. The presence of my love was very important, and JS was, and still is today, perfect in his actions during each cycle. But it should be noted that Sarah helped me a lot in making this process smoother and making me feel less alone. We love our partners dearly, but when among women who inject themselves in the belly, we reach a new level of compassion for each other. We feel less alone, we who live on hormones and freshwater.

Hormones! Let's talk about them! How to drive a woman crazy with just one pill. Oh, sincerely. Let's have a moment of silence for all the women who will have to mentally process these medications, but also for all the men who will have to support their partners with a smile on their faces. Gentlemen, it's not the timc to hold a grudge nor to put the blame on your spouse if you value your life. That's a joke (or not). Some cycles are better than others. We all need time to adapt. A special thanks to my beau for being such an attentive partner!

"One, two, three, twenty-five injections! Seriously, have you seen the number of injections I'm going to have in my belly? It's giving me a panic attack! Look at all the medications I have to take in the coming days! Ready or not, here I go!"

It was the infamous day 1 of the cycle that marked the beginning of the in vitro fertilization process. This day was accompanied by my friend named anxiety, but I kept reminding myself constantly that everything I was doing was for a good cause. I was finally going to have my long-awaited miracle. It was an intense personal journey to undertake, but I was so proud to have come this far. I was ready to do anything to be able to carry a child, and after all that I had already done, it was out of the question to give up now.

May 5, 2022, the day when everything truly began for me. I had to completely destroy this fear from my existence. I had to face the very first injection into my own belly. This one would be given by my partner. One thing at a time, as they say! Mentally, I wasn't ready to give myself this injection, and I also needed my partner to be physically present. After all, we were experiencing this journey together! He had to become a nurse for one evening and even for several more evenings to come, and I clearly had to work on my fear of needles. At exactly 7:00 p.m., it was time! So, I took a deep breath, and we pierced the skin of my belly for the first time. All the while, I was telling myself that it wasn't as hard as I thought it would be. However, from my five-foot vantage point, I could see the pen in Jean-Simon's hands moving in just about every possible direction.

"Gentle, my love, with the pressure, please. I feel like I'm experiencing a huge wave of liquid entering my belly."

"I'm already going gently!"

"Yes, I see that. I don't want to stress you out; just letting you know about my discomfort."

"I understand. I'll be careful, I'm sorry."

"Don't worry, I know it's new for you as well. We can now change careers, you and me! What do you say?"

"Have you lost your mind? Never in a million years! And there goes one. Shall we prepare for the next?"

"Of course! As if one injection per evening wasn't enough. Thanks, infertility!"

It seems I wasn't the only one experiencing stress at this moment. Nevertheless, we were still so happy and, above all, more confident. However, this would be just the first of over a hundred injections to come in my journey. I would become an expert at injections to the point where I preferred to administer them myself because I knew that way, I had full control over the syringe and the desired location in my belly. And God knows I have this bad habit of needing to be in constant control over my existence. Letting go, as they say? I promise you I have plenty of other wonderful qualities, even if fertility gives me more trouble than ever in that regard. Every step, big or small, of this quest, will have allowed me to grow as a woman, in many aspects of my life.

So, breakfast was accompanied by five tablets, lunch by a single one, and supper by two of them. All for about fifteen days. The days of injections, until the egg retrieval, passed by so quickly. Since my body was controlled by medication, my cycle was shorter than the natural cycles experienced during the insemination process. That was a beautiful positive aspect of IVF. I would reach my dream more quickly!

"Okay, my love! I've taken my medication, I'm ready. Now, let's keep our fingers crossed for a good harvest."

Here we are at last, heading towards the biggest step of in vitro fertilization, the egg retrieval. To be honest, I am completely terrified. I'm so scared of the unknown, that I don't even think about the harvest. How many will there be? Will I manage to get embryos? In my mind, the only issue with the retrieval is whether or not it will hurt. I'll have embryos, no matter what!

Thankfully, the sedation worked well on the physical side: zero pain and the feeling that the process lasted for only two minutes. Those are my memories of what I expected to be a huge trauma. However, the call from the clinic the next morning was more difficult to bear than the retrieval itself. In summary, thirteen follicles were observed during the ultrasounds preceding the operation, nine follicles were retrieved, five mature eggs, and finally, two—maybe three—embryos under analysis. These embryos had to prove themselves over the following five days. I was scheduled for an embryo transfer on the exact date of my birthday, May 21st. I received a call every day to give me updates on my babies.

The call on day 3, while I was calmly paddleboarding, felt like a ton of bricks crashing down on me. I was informed that the results of the biopsy done three months earlier had just arrived. The transfer scheduled to take place two days later was canceled. Happy birthday, Virginie. The embryos would have to be frozen. I had just been diagnosed with endometritis, which needed to be treated as it could lead to miscarriage if I were to become pregnant. Jean-Simon looked at me with such sorrow in his eyes. I could see how much he struggled to find the right words. I gathered the little strength I had left in me to paddle back to shore. We remained silent, with only the echo of my tears falling in the river, for sole company. Would I be granted at least one chance soon?

I needed to convince myself that one was better than zero, because ultimately, only one embryo was frozen; the other two unfortunately had ceased to develop before the infamous day 5. The next steps? More medication on the menu! I had to endure a treatment with oral antibiotics, to be taken for two weeks, then undergo another biopsy to ensure that the endometritis is no longer present, and finally wait three months for the transfer of my one and precious frozen embryo.

-"I need positivity right now! I need to take my mind off things. What do you say about an inground pool, my love? Imagine how great it would be for me to be pregnant, splashing around in the pool. Or even with the baby during my maternity leave. We'll be able to make the most of the backyard".

Did I mention that I'm good at getting what I want?

So, we decided to sell the camper to afford a small inground pool. Nothing too big, but enough to make me happy. Sometimes, things just happen at the right time. Three months later, the childhood dream began. It was once again a big project, perfectly timed to keep my mind occupied enough to avoid thinking about the embryo transfer that would take place a few days later. What I didn't know at that moment was that following the transfer and the subcutaneous injections in the buttock, I wasn't allowed baths, let alone the pool. So, I would look at my beautiful pool without being allowed more than dipping my toes in it. Once again, I had to work on my patience. But the best was yet to come.

Many women had a positive test at DPO9! I would surely get a faint line too, finally!!! My first in almost four years of this journey!! I'm going for it.

Nothing. Only a blank test like every other one over the past three years. Unfortunately, our in vitro fertilization ended in failure. Before we started it, Jean-Simon and I had agreed that it would be our very last try, that should it fail, we would stop all our attempts at conceiving. But that was simply impossible. How could I give up after making so many sacrifices, so much effort? I still had six inseminations covered by the health insurance since the arrival of free IVF in Quebec. So, we decided to try inseminations privately! Our doctor suggested a superovulation protocol. With injections of follitropin alfa and letrozole, we aimed for three to four follicles per cycle, which I managed to achieve in each of the three inseminations that followed IVF. Unfortunately, these also ended without a positive result.

"I know it's a lot of money, JS... But I think I want to try IVF one last time. They know better how my body reacts now. After that, we'll stop for good..."

"I agree with you. Just know that you'll always have the final say if you want to stop. It's your body after all, and I know you're doing a lot for us."

Finally, more than 4 years have passed since stopping all contraception. I was patiently waiting for my appointment, with the doctor, scheduled on January 24, 2023. We were going to receive our protocol for this last IVF. It had to be the last one because mentally, I couldn't go on feeling only like a person with infertility. It also represented an amount of over $10,000 that would be spent on this cycle alone. I felt like I was playing at the casino with my money but without the pleasure that comes from it.

On January 26th, my first ultrasound took place to make sure my follicles were ready. The previous appointment coincided very closely with my period. So, we needed to verify if it was possible to start the protocol by skipping the estradiol step. This estrogen hormone is to be taken for about ten days before our periods, and in this case, its function is to mature the follicles while keeping them as close in size as possible. We don't want one follicle to be larger than the others and thus trigger ovulation too early. Fortunately, the follicles were ready! My body was ready! I was ready! Off to the pharmacy to pick up my injections and medication needed to start my cycle. Luckily, injections were no longer a mystery to me. The first one was administered in the car as we left the pharmacy. I was granted a cycle with a good number of injections. How lucky am I! Four injections a day. Phew! But I was prepared to give it my all. I wanted to believe more than ever in this last chance.

"I'm on thirty-six injections, my love. Look at my belly, swollen like never before. I never thought I'd say this, but I'm almost looking forward to the egg retrieval! Three more injections and we finally trigger ovulation!!"

"In any case, your belly gives us a nice preview of what's to come. You'll be a beautiful pregnant woman."

Finally, the day of the retrieval arrived. The stress was at its peak, but it was really different from the first time. I wasn't afraid of the pain. Well, a little bit. I was literally terrified at the thought that none of my eggs would develop into an embryo after fertilization. I couldn't go through the same story again. My mind couldn't handle it. Everything cannot always go wrong, I'm allowed a break every now and then, right? Here I am, lying in the operating room, my arm connected to the sedation.

But I fight. I want to see what happens this time. I want to see the harvest of each one of my follicles. Why is it taking so long? I don't see anything on the screen, and the doctor seems worried. Where are they? There were sixteen of them at the last ultrasound. WHY? No, I can't believe it... OH! THERE THEY ARE! The first three are finally detected. We can finally start breathing again. Oh! And there are more! Barely a few minutes later, the fishing is completed. Finally, more scared than harmed as they say! I had a nice harvest of fifteen eggs. I'm over the moon. But anxiety still manages to get to me. What if none of them develop? What if they're not mature enough after all? I eagerly await the call the next day.

— "Wonderful love of my life whom I love more than anything, could you please go get me a sedative to help me relax, pretty please? (It's always when we're comfortably settled in, that we realize we need something, requiring us to abandon a cozy position we just managed to secure). I'll never be able to close my eyes. This stress gives me incredible nausea, and I hope so much that they'll call me early tomorrow morning. I'm excited, but I'm so scared of what I'm going to hear.

— I'll go. (Preceded by a sigh, clearly filled with love...)

— Thank you, I love you too!

8:26 a.m., the phone rings. It's the embryologist. She eases in the conversation by telling me how she can feel my stress just by hearing my voice. I want to die on the spot and scream at her, "SPIT IT OUT!" Well, sorry! Let's just say that my patience left my body at that moment. So, I make a conscious effort to remain calm and listen attentively, despite the rapid beating of my heart, which is almost deafening and somewhat unsettling.

— "Mme Bisson, I have good news! Out of the fifteen eggs we retrieved, all were mature, and twelve successfully fertilized. We will call you back in two days, on Friday, for another update, and at the same time, I will confirm your appointment on Sunday for the transfer. My heart drops at that moment. I want to cry all the tears of joy from my body, but at the same time, I have my protective shield that refuses to leave my mind. I want to be positive more than ever. I want to believe that this time will finally be my turn, but fear is creeping back in. I'm afraid of hurting so much by believing too much. So, I decided to stay as positive as possible and try to keep my mind occupied for the days to come. Unfortunately, depression managed to take full possession of my body in the days following the retrieval. The buildup of stress, the side effects of certain medications, and once again, this immense fear of repeated failure. I don't think I can stress enough how much my emotional state is like a rollercoaster during this wild journey. One day, I'm filled with more motivation than ever, ready to break down barriers to achieve my miracle. But the next day, I sink into a world that is far too dark to exist. So, I find myself on sick leave, having to take care of my health, but also my body since the transfer is fast approaching.

— I am so happy today, my love! We are going to meet our beautiful 4AA perfect embryo. This is it, this time around! I am also looking forward to knowing how many others will be frozen. I will always remember that perfect smile on my partner's face. He was so happy that we finally reached this point! I saw so much hope and trust in his eyes. We have come a long way since the beginning.

But this time, it was different. Everything was finally going so well. The results of the IVF so far were, for once, so promising. So, we could only believe that it would finally be our turn after all the obstacles we've encountered! It was at that moment that the nurse came to fetch us for this perfect encounter to come. A transfer that went so smoothly, accompanied by several laughs. Now, hold on tight, my darling! Baby is snug and warm, and we are ready to leave the clinic together for our first meal as a family of three. The famous belief says that a good McDonald's would be the winning recipe to help the embryo implant. However, at 9 o'clock in the morning, it might be too early to go eat fries at McDonald's! So, it will be breakfast at a restaurant near the clinic. My body shouldn't notice too much difference between the salty fries from one place or the other. Everything is perfect! But there's always that damned lingering thought that never wants to leave my mind. My mood swings often tend to go from white to black in the blink of an eye. How is it possible to be so happy but also emotionless at the same time? The results have been so beautiful since the beginning of this IVF process, but why would the outcome be different this time for me? I can't repeat it enough, but I'm simply scared. I have four beautiful embryos in the freezer if this transfer doesn't work out. However, will I have the strength to try again and again? My mental health is not at its best, but my head continues to fight in survival mode. I want to keep believing. I deserve this happiness too. Despite all this stress, the infamous day of the blood test arrived quickly enough. The nurse's call followed:

— I'm sorry, Mrs. Bisson. Your blood test is negative. Unfortunately, the embryo did not implant.

As for the next steps, I will need to see the doctor again to receive a new transfer protocol. Why am I not crying? It's as if I'm stepping once again into this same monthly routine to which my entire being is now too accustomed. Failure, sadness, hope, belief, and finally, we start over. Failure, sadness, hope, belief... However, I managed to convince the nurse to contact my assigned doctor for another transfer in the following cycle. Fortunately for me, the doctor agrees to provide me with a new protocol without having to meet me again. I don't have time to dwell on the previous failure. What I'm aiming for is success. However, I must face reality and set limits as our budget is draining faster than it is replenishing. If this transfer turns out to be a failure, I will undergo further tests and request a referral to see another specialist, whom I have only heard reassuring comments about. The wait for an appointment will thus be the enforced halt I must impose on myself. Until then, I pin all my hopes on this transfer which will also happen quite quickly. So, I decide to go all in, into this cycle... As if it wasn't already what I had done in previous attempts... Anyway, let's just say that I googled all the natural products, grandmother's recipes, and other great tricks to accompany me during my third embryo transfer. Thus, our daily menu includes omega-3 capsules, magnesium, and folic acid, raspberry leaf teas, kiwi, quinoa, cashews and also some lovely purple beets that I don't even like. What wouldn't one do to succeed? I cut them into small pieces to make it mentally easier to swallow! I also add guided meditation sessions to my routine using a recommended app that I install on my phone.

I must admit that this app will remain in my daily routine because, for my mental as well as physical well-being, I truly appreciate each ten-minute session of specially designed deep relaxation. With Jean-Simon, we are so confident that this time will be the right one. This transfer cycle has been emotionally charged, and that's an understatement. It took me three ultrasounds before finally getting the green light for a transfer date. As I'm about to leave the room, my doctor walks in. I just saw him a few minutes earlier. My brain immediately switches to stress mode as this is not a common situation.

"Madame Bisson, I've analyzed and recalculated, and ultimately, I want to see you again in three days. Your endometrium could be a little better than today's result, and I would like us to put all the odds in our favor."

I knew I should be happy that he was making sure my body was ready and that we were maximizing all our chances. I was disappointed to once again have an additional delay. What would a fertility process be without delays? Still, the appointment came fairly quickly. I returned to the clinic, but this time alone, thinking it would just be a quick round trip and that my body would certainly be ready. Never in my wildest dreams had my mind considered any unforeseen circumstances. The appointment wasn't with my usual doctor as he wasn't on duty that day.

"I'm sorry, Madame Bisson, but your endometrium hasn't thickened as desired. It's even the opposite. For today, I suggest either to end this transfer or to take five additional days of hormones with increased dosage. I know that mentally, taking medication is challenging, but it might be necessary to adjust our approach."

So, please, get dressed and think about it. You can confirm your decision with the nurse when she calls your name in the waiting room.

I couldn't utter a word. The confusion looping in my head and the tears filling my face prevented me from thinking clearly. Why does it always have to be something negative? Was it possible JUST ONCE to have a cycle where everything went smoothly? I was exhausted from riding the roller coaster. So, I returned to the waiting area, unable to stop my tears, under the questioning gazes I could perceive from each of the women sitting in the room. I just wanted to go hide under the covers of my bed. The room, which appeared quite large at first, seemed to close in on me at that moment. I thought to myself that after taking so many medications, what harm would it do to try five more days, if it meant to give an extra chance to my long-awaited beautiful ending? So, you can imagine that I decided to continue and once again give all my energy, or at least what was left, for this cherished miracle. The third ultrasound came in a snap. I held my breath waiting for the result for this last chance that was being offered to me.

"Madame Bisson, I must confess that the stress is palpable in the room. Haha! You can breathe. Look how beautiful your endometrium is. We will be able to schedule your transfer. Know that it is normal to see variations during its measurements. After all, we measure in millimeters."

I wanted to cry with joy, but my whole body was ready to receive another piece of bad news and remained in defensive mode. Nevertheless, I left the clinic with a tremendous weight off my shoulders. I was so grateful to be able to move forward and be confident with this transfer.

I was sincerely more serene, or rather, less depressed than during previous transfers. I told myself that my body would thank me for being "happier". The day of the transfer arrived so quickly. As much as the delays can seem long in fertility, sometimes each step passes by at the speed of light. The happiness Jean-Simon and I felt was just perfect. The moment was also perfect. I knew the routine well (unfortunately or fortunately). Regardless, we had reached this point and we were so close to our goal (because I knew this time would be the right one). It was my turn! A beautiful 5BA embryo in early expansion was already ready to implant.

I sincerely wished to conclude by announcing that finally, my turn had come after nine inseminations, two egg retrievals, and three embryo transfers. Unfortunately, that won't be today. Perhaps I haven't yet "succeeded" in this aspect of my life, but I swear I haven't said my last word. I am officially on the waiting list for further tests before retrieving my three embryos waiting patiently in storage. I know for sure that one of them will stick. I have to keep believing. I won't hide that this last negative test hurt me a lot at first, but today I'm fine, sincerely. This break allows me to focus on all the other beautiful things around me, and I know that one day I will be the mother of our little mini-us! Until then, my family is expanding in another way. My relatives keep telling me that I'll soon need to get a zoo license. Oops! Let's just say I keep my mind busy with two cats, two dogs, three chickens, and recently, a beautiful saltwater aquarium. Is that called pet therapy? Before I go, I'd like to give you a small piece of advice. Take care of yourself above all else! You are important, and your happiness matters just as much.

You don't define yourself solely as an "infertile woman." I had long forgotten this detail. We are beautiful human beings filled with wonderful qualities, and we will succeed!

CHAPTER 5

ENDOMETRIOSIS, FIBROIDS, SURGERIES, AND RESILIENCE

By Audrey Coutu

Edith, my mother, welcomed me into this world at the age of 34. Throughout my life, I've been reminded time and again that I was a long-awaited, yet unexpected miracle. She married at the tender age of 23, yearning for a family of eight children. However, life took an unexpected turn when a cyst ruptured in her fallopian tube, leading to emergency surgery. The procedure resulted in the removal of one fallopian tube, one ovary, and the diagnosis of endometriosis.

The doctors' verdict was blunt: 'Madam, with your condition, you will never conceive'

You have to know Mom to understand the impact this had on her. She was born to be the mother of a large family. I can now comprehend the shock she must have experienced at such a young age upon learning that her greatest dream would remain unfulfilled. A few years later, she divorced and began her life as a single woman without children. Embracing life, she treated herself to a Corvette, living each day to the fullest. Pouring her passion into her hair salon, she nurtured her career and her business as if it were her child. She passed her passion on to me, and together, we run a thriving family business, source of immense pride for us both.

At the age of 33, against all odds, she defied medical expectations and became pregnant—a miraculous turn of events that left my entire family and my grandmother in disbelief. Love has always been abundant in my life. While my parents parted ways when I was just two years old, my father remained present. Tragically, he succumbed to lung cancer when I turned 22. His calm demeanor and gentle encouragement are sorely missed, particularly during moments of introspection like this.

Strangely, the journey towards fertility brings up many emotions tied to my father's passing. But that's a story for another time."

2010

In my early twenties, at an age when we discover our sexual life, I would feel excruciating pain on the right side of my abdomen, during and after sexual intercourse. At times, the pain was so intense that I struggled to even get out of my car and walk. I would think to myself, "How am I going to pursue a relationship, I'm in so much pain." Imagine talking to my 20-year-old boyfriend, brimming with hormones. I attempted to bring up the subject with him, but at that age, we were both so ignorant about stomach pains and the intricacies of women's bodies. Often, I came across as uninterested, feeling guilty to decline intimacy due to my pain. Nevertheless, we have since reconciled; we were young and poorly educated on the subject. This highlights the importance of keeping an open dialog, enabling young men to comprehend women's bodily ailments and their daily struggles.

Let's get back to my pains, like a big bruise deep in my belly, accompanied by a sense of heaviness radiating down my right leg. It was then that my mother suggested, "I'm sure you have endometriosis like me, ask your doctor." Thus commenced my journey with medical professionals. It was during this period that I realized how enigmatic the female body remained and how often my concerns were dismissed, and still are sometimes. The first doctor I consulted assertively told me: "It's not hereditary, you're too young. We'll do an ultrasound and a scan as a precaution." Yet, nothing abnormal was detected and I was informed it was normal to experience stomach aches and to take ibuprofen as needed.

"If it persists, we'll try switching your contraceptive pill to a stronger one," my doctor told me. Obviously, my pains did not stop. Determined to find answers, my dear mother encouraged me to seek a second opinion, leading to a specialized clinic. I remember the tall doctor who examined me, pressing firmly on my stomach. Though uncomfortable and painful, I was once again dismissed as much too young to have endometriosis. They redirected me to a sex therapist's office, where I found myself with a petite lady armed with pamphlets on pelvic physiotherapy. At 21, I had no idea such treatment existed. The physiologist suggested that my pain might be due to muscle contractions during intercourse and offered help to relax my muscles and manage my pain. Needless to say, I left the clinic. I was in tears, feeling discouraged and misunderstood. 'No,' I thought, 'the pain runs deep in my belly, and I know it's not due to muscle contractions.' I obviously never called her again.

During this period, my father, already battling cancer, received a devastating diagnosis of brain metastases. We braced ourselves for the inevitable. A few months later, I found myself face-to-face with the least friendly gynecologist in town, perhaps even in all of Quebec. I poured my heart out about my pain and my mother's history with endometriosis.

— "Could it be that?"

— "We'll perform a laparoscopy," he declared. "We'll confirm it."

— "A what?"

— "It's a camera that we insert through the stomach to see if you have endometriosis. You'll be under anesthesia, don't worry."

Finally! He might not have been the nicest doctor, but at least, he was taking me seriously. I owe it to my mom for urging me to consider endometriosis as a possible cause. Without her support and guidance, I might never have received a diagnosis.

Despite all this, I constantly doubt: "Maybe the pain is all in my head. Maybe I don't need to take this test after all." Truth be told, I wasn't too keen about it.

NOVEMBER 2010

The night before my surgery, I stayed at my mother's house. My father wished to accompany me as well, but his health was deteriorating and mobility was becoming a challenge. So, despite his desire, it was my loving mother who stood by my side, understanding the depths of my struggle all too well, having endured similar pains in her youth. As I faced my first ever surgery under anesthesia, apprehension crept in. The thought of undergoing abdominal surgery stirred anxiety within me, prompting thoughts of cancelling it altogether. I couldn't shake the fear of inconveniencing doctors and nurses, for what might turn out to be nothing. But soon, the doctor arrived, ready to escort me to the operating room. Alone, I lay on the stretcher, unable to be accompanied by my mother any further. Navigating through a corridor filled with patients awaiting their turn for surgery, I felt isolated. Once on the operating table, a small oxygen mask was placed over my face. In mere seconds, I drifted into a blissful oblivion. An hour later, I emerged from the anesthesia, the haze of sedation slowly dissipating.

I wasn't too young, nor was I imagining my pain, and pelvic physiotherapy was not what I needed. The diagnosis was clear—endometriosis. The surgeons meticulously removed particles from my bladder and addressed the source of my persistent pain on the right side."

DECEMBER 2010

It was at the same time that I found myself navigating the challenging journey of accompanying my father through his illness. Having never remarried, he now found himself alone, in the realm of palliative care. As his only child, the responsibility of deciding to transfer him to the Rosemont center for end-of-life care rested solely on my shoulders. We were given a timeline: three months, perhaps even less. I made it a point to visit him at the hospital three, four times a week, often finding myself alone, in his company. Together, we shared beautiful moments, watching movies and indulging in pizza, hoping for a miraculous recovery while simultaneously longing for an end to his suffering. Each day brought its load of emotions, as I juggled the responsibilities of caring for Chico, his beloved dog, tending to his house, and preserving his cherished guitars.

A noteworthy anecdote comes to mind: Upon receiving his cancer diagnosis, my father resolved to reignite his passion for music. He joined a music group and even graced the stage with two concerts in the years leading up to his passing. His enthusiasm knew no bounds, evident in his collection of forty guitars—yes, you read that right, forty guitars! He was like a teenager reliving his youth. Music and concerts have always held a significant place in my life; beautiful memories that I cherish dearly. My father, a dentist and orthodontist, was a man of passion, often living life unconventionally. His 'live and let live' attitude brought me comfort.

MARCH 2011

On March 1st, 2011, I bid farewell to my father. As I reflect on those times now, at the age of 34, I realize the weight of the burden I carried at such a tender age. I had just broken up with my boyfriend at the time. All my friends were living their best lives with the carefree attitude of their twenties. I was emptying out my father's closets all alone in his big house. Unknowingly, it was going to give me strength of character, a resilience that continues to help me today. As the months passed, the pain persisted in my abdomen. Adhesions, maybe? Hormonal treatments were prescribed to me as a precautionary measure against the looming threat of endometriosis.

It consisted in a monthly painful injection on the buttock, for nine months. It induced an artificial menopause and helped reduce the inflammation of endometriosis. As a result, side effects started to affect me: menopausal heat waves, losing my hair, mood swings ... Pure happiness, right?!

As an only child, I always had a fascination with big families and action-filled family reunions. I love entertaining and cooking. All my life, I have imagined myself in the middle of a large table filled with children... friends of my children... Our friends and those of our parents. In short, I love entertaining and cooking. It's a nice way to show people that I love them. It may sound crazy, but I dream of making lunches and cooking meals every week for my children.

2018

A little jump in time.

It's towards the end of 2017, when I was 29, that serendipity led me to encounter the love of my life at a local bar. Meeting him felt like a beautiful gift from the universe. It was like a scene, straight out of a romantic movie. Ours is a love that feels pure, wholesome, and utterly unique— a once-in-a-lifetime kind of love. Unbeknownst to us, we had grown up in the same city, only two kilometers apart and shared several acquaintances. Quickly, we moved in together, discussing dreams of matrimony and parenthood. Wrapped in a cocoon of happiness, I knew deep within my heart that he was the one I had been waiting for. In that moment, I felt an overwhelming sense of gratitude towards life itself.

2020

In February 2020, at the beginning of my 31st year, just before the COVID pandemic, we decided that I'd stop taking the birth control pill and to venture into the realm of parenthood. Amongst my close circle of friends, I was the first to take this leap of faith. Little did I know that, three years down the line, while my friends would be welcoming one or two bundles of joy into their lives, my own journey would be filled with challenges.

As the months passed, my health began to falter, marked by increasingly prolonged and agonizing menstrual cycles. The joyous news of my friends' pregnancies weighed on me and I found myself longing for my turn.

-"It's normal, these things take time", my mother would reassure me, repeating that if she managed to get pregnant, the same thing would eventually happen to me. I wanted to believe her, but a sense of unease lingered. What's peculiar about this journey is not knowing what awaits us and praying to avoid the fate of those for whom conception remains elusive. To be in constant anticipation of something that doesn't happen, month after month.

With the best intentions, everyone tries to be comforting.

— *"I'm sure it's coming! My friend's friend got pregnant just before her first fertility appointment.*

— My sister stopped thinking about it, and it worked after a year and a half.

— Do it every other day.

— Do it every day.

— Have you tried acupuncture or naturopathy?

— Stress isn't good, you know?

— My niece got pregnant after six years, so anything is possible.

— You're healthy, you're young, you have time.

— Women have children later now. You're not alone.

— Yes, it took me a long time as well. It took me nine months...

— You never know. I might have difficulties for my second...

I heard them all and each time someone offers one of these well-meaning phrases, I feel the urge to respond sharply. I feel like my distress isn't being heard or acknowledged. Because, no, the path to conception isn't paved with wishful thinking alone. I understand that people intend to offer empathy, but the reality is, many simply don't comprehend the depths of infertility. I often sense the apprehension in others' eyes, the fear of walking in my shoes, especially when a mere three months of trying yield no positive results. In those moments, I find myself offering reassurances, assuring them that it's normal, that conception may take up to a year without any underlying issues. More often than not, they find success in the ensuing months. However, the only reality my boyfriend and I have is that none of these words of encouragement or advice apply to us right now.

2021

As I sat in the gynecologist's office, the very one who, despite his shortcomings, had always taken my concerns seriously from the beginning, despite my young age, I found myself grappling with a mix of emotions. In June, as we crossed the one-year mark of trying to conceive, I asked for a fertility referral, alongside addressing my excruciatingly heavy and painful periods.

During the examination, he pressed my abdomen both internally and externally, causing discomfort that had become all too familiar. With a solemn expression, he delivered the news, 'It appears that the endometriosis has returned. There's little I can offer in terms of treatment, aside from medication. However, it will reduce your chances of conceiving due to its side effects. You could still take them until your fertility appointment.'

It was a pivotal moment as the notion of in vitro fertilization (IVF) was introduced for the first time. Research indicated that women with endometriosis often turned to IVF. Faced with the prospect of enduring months of futile attempts, I made the difficult decision to forego the medication, opting instead to start fertility procedures.

Reflecting back, I couldn't help but wonder if things might have been different had I chosen to alleviate my pain temporarily with medication. If only I had known then what I know now...

At the time, little did I know that my symptoms weren't solely attributed to endometriosis. As I began making calls, I quickly realized that every clinic, whether public or private, had months-long waiting lists. The frustration was palpable as I faced the reality of six-month waits for appointments. What I had hoped would be a visit scheduled for the following week turned into a waiting game extending for months.

As time wore on, my symptoms exacerbated. My periods became increasingly debilitating, marked by excessive bleeding and excruciating pain. One September evening, curled up in a warm bath, I turned to my partner and voiced my growing concern:

— "Honey, something doesn't feel right. I'm convinced it's more than just endometriosis. The level of pain I'm experiencing is far from normal. I fear it might be something as serious as cancer."

I've always experienced stomach pain, but recently, my periods have become unbearable. They disrupt my daily life entirely. I constantly find myself staining my underwear, pants, and even my sheets. I rely on XL tampons and pads, yet they overflow three times a day. My periods drag on for eight days, followed by light bleeding and mild cramps until the twentieth day of my cycle. I'm left with just five days to attempt to return to my normal routine of training and socializing. During those 5 days, it's almost as if I forget the extent of my suffering: 'There, I'm getting back on track.'

But deep down, I know it's not that simple. I can't control my body's response, and I constantly blame myself for not being strong enough to endure the pain and bleeding. I'm forced to cancel dinners and scale back on the physical activities that once brought me so much joy. As a result, I've gained weight, and my stomach is so bloated that I can't even see my feet in the shower. The constant bloating leaves me looking as though I'm pregnant.

"I absolutely must shed this weight before considering pregnancy,' I tell myself, falling into a cycle of obsessive weighing and fluctuating weight. I lose five pounds during the week, only to regain them over the weekend. Insomnia plagues me as I struggle with discomfort in my own body. I no longer recognize myself in the mirror, feeling ugly and fat, which further lowers my spirits."

My self-esteem takes a nosedive. I wear loose clothing in an attempt to conceal my weight gain. I've always been fit, and for me, it's very disconcerting to experience the way others now perceive my body; a body that seems to have a mind of its own, one that I no longer recognize or love. I start to feel less mentally alert and tired.

In October, we finally received a call from a clinic. Our initial consultation with our doctor takes place over the phone due to COVID-19 restrictions. We need to undergo basic tests including blood tests, ultrasound, and a semen analysis. Considering my endometriosis, our doctor advises us to consider IVF. Fortunately, the free first cycle is coming into effect at the same time. However, our doctor tells us to await the results of the basic tests before making any firm plans.

It's fall. I'm thinking "If everything goes well, I'll start treatment in January 2022 and I'll be pregnant in February or March. YES! It'll go fast, I can't wait!" Boy! I was naive and I didn't know what we were getting ourselves into.

On December 20th, we have the follow-up call. That's when I hear about fibroids. I'm also told that the tube on my right side seems blocked. My bleeding isn't normal either.

Uh oh!

If I decide to treat the blocked tube, I would be subjected to a painful test, a risk of infection related to endometriosis, and several months of waiting. So, we elected to proceed with the initial plan, as recommended by my doctor. We'll have a hysteroscopy and an endometrial biopsy in March to comprehend the reason for my heavy bleedings. We're moving forward. I'm on the waiting list for IVF. The next available slots are in April.

"April?! That's so far away!"

The disappointment cuts deep. Patience will be necessary. While waiting for April, I have to take medication for three months, to alleviate the symptoms of endometriosis.

— "Conceiving naturally during this period could result in an ectopic pregnancy. These are the potential side effects of the medication", I'm cautioned.

Another blow to the heart. It dawns on me that I won't have a baby in 2022. I tell myself that at least I'll be pregnant by next Christmas, and then I'll give birth in 2023...

Here we stand on December 23, 2021. Just two days after receiving our test results, my period arrives, making its unwelcome appearance during the holiday season. On Christmas Eve, with my mother and my in-laws visiting, I struggle to navigate through the day. To endure the pain, I find myself needing to take ibuprofen every four hours. The cramps are so severe, I can even feel them in my jaw. This has undoubtedly been one of the toughest times yet. Just before dinner, waves of nausea wash over me, accompanied by more excruciating stomach pain. I retreat to the bathroom, replenish my ibuprofen supply, and swap out my saturated sanitary pad and tampon for the third time that day. Gazing at myself in the mirror, I offer words of encouragement, but still, a few tears of frustration manage to escape. With a deep breath, I collect myself and return to the evening's festivities.

The anti-inflammatories finally kick in. I feel the energy slowly returning, allowing me to engage with my guests. However, as I bid farewell to my family and rise from my chair, I suddenly feel something wet. Panic sets in as I realize my hand is covered in blood. My tampon has overflowed, staining my pad and soaking through my tights. There's even blood on the bench. I'm in so much pain that night that I only managed to sleep a few hours.

The same scenario repeats the next day, during the bacon-wrapped sausage feast, at the Christmas dinner. I find myself spending the night on the couch, unable to escape the pain. The next day, everything is stained with blood: my pajamas, the sheets, even the bathroom floor when I go to the toilet in the morning.

Quite charming, isn't it?

2022

Apart from the grief of losing my father, this has been the most challenging year of my life. I never imagined I could experience such intense pain and conflicting emotions. It's as if, in that year, emotions I had buried for a decade had suddenly resurfaced. It feels like such an injustice! Why is it always me facing these difficult times? My early twenties were marked by my father's passing, and now, in my thirties, I'm grappling with infertility. I have no choice, it's my journey. I know there are worse things on Earth, but deep down, I find it really unfair and hard to accept. The isolation, the loneliness, the changing dynamics of friendships; it feels like my life is at a standstill. I understand that everyone faces their own challenges, but when you experience the death of a loved one, illness, or infertility, the sense of solitude can be overwhelming.

People move on with their lives, and I'm left feeling like the world keeps spinning while I'm stuck in my pain. I'm fortunate to have my boyfriend, who has become my anchor through this storm. My mother's unconditional support is also a source of strength. Without them, I don't know how I would have made it through this ongoing turmoil.

JANUARY 2022

Let's rewind to the moment when I first started taking the medication. Swallowing that first pill felt like a weight in my mouth, a reminder of the daunting journey ahead: "One down, eighty-three to go...." That's when it gets tricky. In the initial month, the bleeding was relentless. Clots became a daily occurrence, as if I were enduring heavy periods that refused to cease. Concerned, I reached out to the clinic multiple times, seeking reassurance. Their response was simple: endure and persist.

After two months, the bleeding finally subsided, but in its wake came overwhelming fatigue. My energy levels plummeted, disrupting my usual workout routine. Despite this struggle, my weight remained unchanged, and I felt increasingly dissatisfied with my appearance. None of my clothes fit anymore, and I couldn't shake the feeling of being unattractive. Even when my boyfriend assured me of my beauty, I found it difficult to love myself. Navigating my depression was challenging for both of us. Though our relationship remained strong, my boyfriend often felt helpless in the face of my struggles. Despite the difficulties, we found moments of laughter and connection amidst the turmoil.

Fast forward to March, the day of the hysteroscopy and biopsy. Anxiety skyrocketed as I anticipated the pain. Unfortunately, my doctor's COVID-19 diagnosis meant I wouldn't meet her in person. Another doctor stepped in, opting to proceed with only the biopsy due to concerns about infection. Her cautionary tale of a patient's complication during a similar test solidified my decision to follow her advice. Though the biopsy was uncomfortable, lasting only about 10 seconds, it revealed a new piece of the puzzle: my hydrosalpinx tube.

— "Huh? I was never told that!

— When liquid is found in the tube, we call it hydrosalpinx.

— Okay, but I thought it was just blocked. I've read about failed transfers with hydrosalpinx tubes. Why wasn't I told about this before?

— If there's no fluid in the uterus, we're not immediately worried. Sometimes, when there are one or two failed transfers, we can have the tube removed, but that's six months to a year of waiting. We're not there yet."

Leaving the clinic, tears blur my vision, my heart heavy from what I've just been told. Thoughts of the looming six to twelve months of waiting and potential embryo failures echo in my mind. I weep all the way home, seeking a bit of comfort on my couch.

Three months have passed. I can finally stop my medication. My periods return with a vengeance: heavy, prolonged and excruciating.

April marks the commencement of my IVF journey. My biopsy reports no alarming findings. Graced with a six-week protocol, I brace myself for all the hormones and injections to come; forty in total. I decided to trust my medical team, thinking this protocol was selected because of my endometriosis.

I am prepared—or so I tell myself. Months of consultations with a psychologist and the practice of positive visualization have equipped me as best they could. The protocol unfolds: three weeks of oral hormones followed by three weeks of injections. The first three weeks were the toughest for my body. Quickly, I start feeling the side effects. I have dreadful bleeding, blood clots, unlike anything I've ever experienced. I don't have severe period pain, but I really don't feel well. Once again, I stain all my clothes.

I recall one morning when even the smallest tasks felt like monumental challenges. As I stepped out of the shower to prepare for work, I found myself confronted with a scene straight out of a nightmare. Blood had seeped into my slippers, and I could feel it pooling around my ankles. In that moment of distress, my boyfriend returned from his walk, and I called out to him for help.

Returning to the shower, I felt not just discouraged but completely drained by the relentless bleeding. Despite reaching out to my clinic multiple times over the past weeks, I received the same reassurance: it was rare, but it could happen, and I should carry on.

During this tumultuous time, I faced two options each day. I could either retreat to my couch, feeling utterly depleted, or summon every ounce of strength to navigate through my workday in survival mode, despite the overwhelming fatigue.

One particular morning, the decision whether to cancel my workday loomed heavily. Yet, I reasoned with myself that perhaps stepping out of the house would offer a bit of a break. However, rescheduling client appointments became increasingly challenging, as the uncertainty of my next fertility appointments loomed large.

As I left for work, my bag weighed down with ibuprofen, tampons, and pads, I braced myself for the day ahead. Welcoming my client at the salon, I couldn't help but catch a glimpse of my reflection in the mirror.

"OMG! I am pale and green," I muttered to myself, a reminder of the toll this relentless ordeal had taken on me.

I decided to return home and cancel the rest of the day. Both my body and mind had reached their limits. Adding to the weight of my burden, throughout this journey, several of my clients had shared their joyful news of pregnancy. Each announcement is a bittersweet reminder of the unpredictable nature of my own journey. While I genuinely share in their happiness, I can't help but feel the pang of longing and uncertainty that accompanies my own path.

The second phase begins and I'm ready to start the injections. Gradually, my bleeding calms down. On the morning of the first injection, I am filled with motivation, but totally scared at the same time. My boyfriend has made a playlist of soft songs, creating an atmosphere reminiscent of a scene from "This Is Us." Despite the preparation, I find myself hesitating for long minutes before finally mustering the courage to administer the syringe near my navel. Though it's not a significant shot, the task looms large, especially at 7:30 in the morning. Tears well up as I complete the injection, a mixture of nervousness, relief, and pride washing over me. With each subsequent injection, the process becomes a bit easier to handle. At one point, I found myself needing to administer hormones three times a day. Simultaneously, I try to live my life as normally as possible, but my mind isn't fully present. Fatigue begins to take its toll.

The day of the egg retrieval finally arrives. Following the hormone intake, a lengthy needle is inserted through the vaginal route to extract as many mature eggs as possible. My boyfriend stands by my side during the procedure, wearing his cute hospital "shower cap." Though I can't see him, his comforting small talk about our dog and his reassuring touch on my hand provide solace. Despite the anesthesia, I keenly feel the needle piercing my belly, causing me to squirm uncomfortably. The medical team increases my dosage in an effort to alleviate the pain, but it persists. Despite my efforts to relax, I reach a breaking point. Every person responds differently, and for me, the retrieval process was excruciatingly painful.

The result: sixteen eggs are successfully retrieved.

The nurses tell me, "Wow, that's a really good result!" Hearing their words fills me with joy, yet I know deep down, it's a little more complex. I'll undergo a frozen embryo transfer because I'm at risk of hyperstimulation. I leave the clinic with my transfer schedule, planned for early July. Today is May 23rd.

Each passing day feels like an eternity, plagued by bleeding, waiting, and stress. It's a concoction that threatens to unravel my sanity and well-being.

For those familiar with the process, waiting for the embryo count is as nerve-wracking as awaiting the transfer result. Typically, the average number of fertilized embryos ranges from three to four. However, outcomes vary widely—some individuals receive a bounty of eight or nine embryos, while others are less fortunate, obtaining only one or none. Predictions are elusive; hope becomes our sole companion.

Then comes the call from the embryologist on the second day post-retrieval.

— "Hello, out of sixteen, we have fertilized eleven. That's an excellent result, Mrs. Coutu.

— Do you think I'll end up with more than three in the end?

— There's a good chance."

Filled with hope, I announce the encouraging news to my boyfriend.

Another call came in on the fifth day post-retrieval. I'm very battered from the retrieval. My belly is swollen. I suffer from constipation, and my periods are about to start again.

The phone rings.

— "Hello, Mrs. Coutu. I don't have very good news. You've lost several of the eleven fertilized embryos. We'll only be able to freeze two out of the eleven. With a bit of luck, there might be a third one tomorrow."

Another blow to the heart. A real one. I still remember the pain of writing the number two on a piece of paper.

I called my partner at work. Without hesitation, he left work and came rushing home. Devastated with this news, both of us started crying. The previous call had given us so much hope. We took a moment to reflect and realized we had no other options but to move forward. Two embryos were better than none. If needed, we were prepared to start the whole process again. After all, as the saying goes, it only takes one.

That evening, we had plans to attend a show with friends. I tried to weigh the pros and cons, then I decided to go. It turned out to be a lesson of self-awareness; I should have stayed home. Learning to set boundaries and tune into my needs has been an essential part of this process. We learn as we go, sometimes through trial and error. I spent half of Charlotte Cardin's show outside the venue. I felt nauseous and had hot flashes, right in the heart of Montreal's busy Ste-Catherine Street. I felt bad for my partner. He missed the entire show because of me. I remained silent all night. I was just a shadow of myself... I felt dead inside and physically, I felt like my stomach was going to explode.

The next day, the phone rings.

— "Yes, hello, Mrs. Coutu. I'm calling to let you know that we froze another embryo today.

— So, do we have three? Is the last one good? Is it of good quality?

— Of course.

— Okay, bye!"

Each time, the calls last less than two minutes. The most stressful two minutes in the world.

Well. Three is better than two. We feel relieved, but I'm still sad about the result. The same emotion as a heartbreak. It hurts for a long time, but a little less each day.

Looking back, I'm very happy to have had three beautiful embryos. Yet, in that moment, I was still in shock from the roller coaster of emotions I had just endured. Anxiety doesn't dissipate with the snap of a finger; its shadow lingers. As anticipated, my period arrives, at the beginning of June, as painful and heavy as it was before my hormone treatments. This time, however, the bleeding persists longer than usual.

I called the clinic and they told me, "If you're still bleeding in a week, call us back."

Obviously, I'm still bleeding a week later. What a surprise...

This is when my journey took an unexpected turn.

After an ultrasound it's determined that a hysteroscopy is necessary to investigate my uterine cavity, a test overlooked in March. My bleeding is abnormal. At best, they might find a removable polyp. At worst, a fibroid. The timeline to address a fibroid varies from six months to a year. As the doctor keeps telling me, "We're not there yet." Then, the verdict arrives in early July. I have two fibroids. One that is fully within my uterine cavity and the other that is halfway in the cavity. At last, an explanation for my pain and bleeding emerges. Removing the fibroids offers hope for pain relief. However, implanting an embryo amidst fibroids poses a heightened risk of miscarriage, prompting a halt in the fertility process. I must undergo fibroid removal at a different hospital, putting my embryo transfer on indefinite hold. With my partner at work, my mother accompanies me. I'm in disbelief; the embryo transfer is on hold…

Now, I must await the surgery timeline, realizing my stomach pains will persist until then. Discouraged, all I yearn for is to reclaim my vitality, my health, and ultimately, the chance to have a baby.

A colleague gynecologist from my fertility doctor's office is supposed to call me within the week. For seven consecutive nights, tears flood my pillow, and each day's commute to work becomes a battleground of emotions. It's summer, I'm supposed to enjoy my new home and life. I have everything to be happy, but I hurt so much inside. I tell myself it's not a life-threatening illness, others have it worse.

Meanwhile, there are constant pregnancy announcements from our friends. We celebrate their joy wholeheartedly, yet deep down, I hurt every time. Witnessing my partner's breakdown after one such announcement is a heart-wrenching moment. Though it pains me to see him in such distress, his vulnerability becomes a catalyst for my own strength. In his tears, I feel like I find the strength to support him. I love him so much that his pain resonates within me, feeling what he feels when he sees me in pain.

On July 13, we're hosting a gathering at our home. Hosting has always been a source of joy for me, especially when it's a celebration for my partner. Our home is filled with the laughter of our friends and the playful energy of eleven children running around the house and the yard. Each of our friends has one, two, or even three children of their own.

As the evening progresses, another couple among our friends shares their exciting news: they're expecting a baby. Despite my genuine happiness for them, I can't help but feel a pang of bittersweet emotion. It's become a habit, almost a ritual, to observe who's drinking and who's not at the start of such gatherings. In moments like these, my heart swells with joy for our friends, I don't wish anyone to endure the same struggles we're facing.

The evening passes, it's really a beautiful day. I finally managed to clear my mind because we have such great friends. It's not seeing children that hurts me, but more the announcement of pregnancies, because this is what I wish to experience for myself, not to have other people's children.

The next morning, and for the first time, I see my partner cry because an event and an announcement hit him hard. I open my eyes and I see his saddest look ever. We talked about it for hours, and I realized that he's feeling the same pain I've been carrying for months now. Quickly, he brushes it off, but it broke my heart to see him like this. Finally, I muster the words, a cliché that I've come to loathe: "It will be okay." Surprisingly, instead of sinking deeper into despair, we find ourselves sharing a laugh. It's then that I understood the innate tendency to utter this phrase to those we hold dear, in moments of comfort.

The week passes by, still without a call from the doctor who is supposed to perform the operation. Armed only with the name of the hospital and his name, I called the central office, hoping for a breakthrough. I call him every day for a week, without success.

By Friday, my frustration boils over, bursting into tears on the phone, I beg the secretary for some reassurance. Finally, a bit of hope emerges: an appointment for a consultation on July 25th. Relief washes over me, and for the first time in two weeks, I drift off to sleep without crying. Through this storm, I'm thankful that fate has led me to such a kind and compassionate gynecologist. I think he understood the urgency and my distress.

The surgery is scheduled for August 13th. What a relief, when I was bracing myself for a possible delay of up to a year! As the days crept closer, a new hurdle emerged: a mandatory COVID-19 test. A positive result would spell out a six-week setback. On August 8th, my partner, battling a minor cold, decided to take the test. As I anxiously awaited the outcome, I glimpsed at the result before he did. "Dan!!! You're positive!"

What are the odds? A positive COVID-19 test. We can't believe it! This is so typical of the luck we've had so far; complications seemed to find their way to us, as if they were drawn to our doorstep.

In the end, no harm was done, as he didn't transmit the virus to me. Luck is finally on our side. The surgery proceeded smoothly, offering a glimmer of hope. After the operation, I had to put the fertility process on hold for six weeks. During this mandatory break, I gradually felt a weight lifting off my shoulders, slowly finding myself again. My stomach pains have decreased a lot; I could now manage with just a pad or tampon, without experiencing any overflow. It was surreal to experience normal periods. At that moment, I realized the extent of my illness over the past two years. Despite the improvement, I still experienced discomfort and occasional pains on my right side.

In September 2022, after nearly a year of fertility treatments, I will finally undergo my first embryo transfer. The ultrasounds leading up to it are nerve-wracking. We still observe a portion of the fibroid remaining, but I'm reassured that it shouldn't re-enter my uterine cavity too quickly. The issue with my hydrosalpinx tube is mentioned every time I have my periods. However, in the ultrasound just before the transfer, we see that the fibroid is no longer in my cavity, and the inflammation in my tube has decreased. With the doctor's green light, I can now schedule my transfer.

The big day arrives!

A few days earlier, a client told me that the doctors dropped her niece's embryo on the floor before her transfer.

"But why are you telling me this?!" I think to myself. I didn't even know it could happen.

During the fertility process, the medical staff keeps telling me how bad stress is.

"How can I tell you this? It's physically and mentally impossible not to be stressed and just be relaxed like on any other day. "

Breathing techniques, yoga, walking, hot baths, reading, paint by numbers, cooking, puzzles, dinners with friends. I DID EVERYTHING. I consulted. Hypnosis was the last stress-relieve option I had not tried yet. With this first transfer, it is also the first time I have to experience the agony of waiting for a test result. After the transfer was done, we decided to go out for breakfast. I feel confident and excited at the same time. My in-laws are nervous and impatient. My mother is holding her breath.

Three days after my transfer, I experienced a sharp pain on my right side, reminiscent of the pain I often endure during my cycles, which I attribute to endometriosis. That's when I lost control. I was taken aback by the anxiety that consumed me during those eleven days leading up to the blood test. The test would confirm whether I was pregnant or if I would need to undergo a second embryo transfer. The waiting was excruciating.

On the morning of the eleventh day, we headed to the clinic for the anticipated blood test. After a few minutes, we returned home... to wait. The ensuing hours felt interminable as we paced around the house, awaiting a call that could alter the course of our lives. "We will call you between 1 pm and 6 pm," we were informed.

17:45, the phone rings: "Hello Audrey! How are you? Unfortunately, it's negative. You can stop taking your hormones and schedule an appointment with your doctor. Have a good evening."

That was it. The entire phone conversation. After a heavy silence, my partner and I break down in tears. These are intense tears, tears that are rarely shed in a lifetime. We seek solace with our parents, knowing they share in our disappointment and are eagerly awaiting the joy of becoming grandparents. We had planned to share the good news with them that same evening, accompanied by our beloved dog. I had envisioned myself pregnant by Christmas... After all we've been through, I feel consumed by anger.

Meanwhile, I take out the ovulation tests and start over again, hoping to regain some semblance of control over my journey to conception. Those who have endured years of trying understand how fertility struggles can alter intimacy. With the bleeding, stomach pains, anxiety, and fatigue, it's been a quieter and very different year in that regard. I started blaming myself for not doing enough, for not being proactive earlier. Little did I know that stopping progesterone would halt my menstrual cycle altogether. The following month, our timing was completely off. A 45-day cycle left me clinging to false hopes of pregnancy, only to realize that I had miscalculated everything. The guilt weighed heavily on me."

I mentioned earlier that luck hasn't exactly been on our side, as evidenced by the COVID-19 incident just before my surgery.

Well, our streak of unfortunate events continued. After our only month of natural trying in a year, I ended with a Bartholin's gland cyst. It's a small, hard bump that develops at the entrance of the vagina, resulting from a rarely blocked gland. Typically, it requires draining due to infection, causing considerable pain."

-"Babe, guess what? I have a Bartholin's cyst. I have to take sitz baths two, three times a day to reduce it and hope it doesn't get infected."

"Are you serious? I don't know what to say anymore because you're so unlucky."

"I know it sounds like a bad joke. Can you go to the pharmacy and buy me a nice sitz bath and some salts? I don't know what it looks like, I can't help you."

He comes back with the equipment. I fill my new friend with warm water and salts and then sit my lady parts in it. I think it's unreal. I start to laugh. Eventually, the cyst goes away on its own after two weeks.

The holidays are approaching, and I desperately need a break. It seems like every month of this year has brought its share of bad news. I can't help but hope that the coming year will be kinder to us.

JANUARY 2023

The year begins and I'm certain that by next Christmas, I'll be cradling my baby in my arms. The holiday season was particularly challenging for me as I continued to mourn the loss of my embryo. I'm exhausted, unable to maintain my usual work pace with the appointments and fertility treatments. I decided to cut back my work hours by one day. The weeks pass by. Slowing down is good for me.

LATE FEBRUARY

The moment arrives for our second embryo transfer, five months after our initial disappointment. Time seems to stretch endlessly as we witness the passing of months and seasons. We wait... and wait... and wait. The ultrasound procedure precedes the second transfer, and once again, the doctor brings up the familiar topics of the fibroid and my hydrosalpinx tube. It feels like déjà vu, the story repeating itself once more.

At my clinic, I rarely see the same doctor, so once again, I find myself recounting my medical history, emphasizing that the surgery successfully removed the fibroid from my uterine cavity. The doctor, now reassured, advises me to begin hormone therapy and return the following Monday. As I depart, tears well up yet again, triggered by a post-traumatic shock induced by the tumult my body has endured over the past year. Surprisingly, it's not the fibroid that preoccupies my mind, as my gynecologist assured me it wouldn't re-enter my cavity too quickly. Instead, it's my tube that unnerves me more than usual.

Fibroids, hydrosalpinx tubes, endometriosis, risk of ectopic pregnancy. It's all swirling in my head, and I can't help the rising anxiety rule over me.

MARCH 2023

The following Monday, our world crumbles yet again. During my last ultrasound before the transfer, I find myself in a familiar room with two English-speaking doctors. They conduct the ultrasound and once again bring up my fibroid. Irritated, I reiterate what I explained to their colleagues just the week before. However, both seem quite concerned and mention that it appears a fibroid has returned to my cavity. I spot my primary doctor walking down the hall. I ask if it's possible to speak with her. The two doctors, still looking worried, continue the conversation, undisturbed. While I'm proficient in English, I reach a breaking point and need to talk about my medical condition in French to make sure I comprehend the importance and the meaning of everything that is being stated. I catch a snippet of their conversation mentioning "both hydrosalpinx," but they quickly return to discussing my fibroid, and my tubes are not mentioned again.

As one of the doctors fetches my primary physician, tears silently stream down my cheeks while I lie there with the ultrasound wand between my legs. The room fills with a sense of urgency as my doctor arrives, accompanied by her colleagues. They huddle together, exchanging murmurs, and the gravity of the situation becomes palpable. It's confirmed—a part of the fibroid is indeed encroaching into my uterine cavity. Even a seasoned colleague is summoned for a second opinion, adding to the intensity of the moment. Amidst the whirlwind of medical discussion, one of them offers a gentle reassurance, stroking my hair and soothing my worries about the upcoming procedure.

My doctor, pressed for time, hastily sends a text to the gynecologist who previously operated on me, seeking guidance on my complex case. Meanwhile, the ultrasound expert delivers the sobering news: it would be unwise to proceed with the embryo transfer given the current circumstances. Perhaps this setback will allow us to fully remove the fibroid, potentially improving our chances of success.

In the midst of it all, I'm struck by the empathy and compassion in their eyes. Though routine for them, each doctor in the room shares a common goal—to navigate this challenging journey with me and to help fulfill my deepest desire of conceiving.

I cry. "It can't be! I just got an operation for the same reason!"

They explain to me that the fibroid may have grown, possibly due to the hormones I've been taking. Overwhelmed with emotion, I broke down in tears, with such intensity, they decided to call my partner from the waiting room. My sobs echo through the corridors. As I emerge from the examination room, I clutch in my hand a business card of a psychologist and a printout of the ultrasound image, resembling those cherished during pregnancy—only this time, it's a blurry depiction of a fibroid.

The pain is overwhelming... Once again, everything comes to a standstill. I cried so much that night that my ribs hurt for three days afterwards. I have headaches and I'm exhausted. I've made the decision to undergo the removal of one of my tubes, hoping to alleviate some of the uncertainties that have plagued me from the start. I feel at loss. I had envisioned this summer with such clarity, picturing myself in a beige dress, pregnant and radiant. It may sound silly, but I had immersed myself in positive visualization, envisioning a future where I'd be pregnant and blissfully happy. I had set milestones in my mind—hoping to give birth before my 35th birthday, believing it would somehow ease the pressure of crossing that threshold. I had convinced myself that by next Christmas, I'd be cradling my newborn, and we'd all rejoice in the miracle. But now, I must come to terms with the fact that 2023 will not be the year I become a mother, nor will I beat the ticking clock of 35. I'm often reminded, "It's okay, age doesn't matter. It'll keep you young. Nowadays, women have children at 40." But I've been on this journey since I was 31. I'm slowly seeing my thirties slip away. Even though I want to enjoy life, the process is so difficult that it consumes me every day.

And so, we left the clinic, having halted our treatment. We had arrived in separate cars for the ultrasound, my partner needing to rush to work afterward. He seemed more tense than usual this time, and in the end, his apprehension was valid. Together, we sit in my car, enveloped in shared sorrow. I look at him, questioning if he's done with the process, if he wants to continue. I can't shake the feeling of responsibility for his sadness; after all, it's my body that seems to be the obstacle. While we know his sperm is somewhat affected, it's not enough to prevent a natural pregnancy.

In short, it's my damn belly that's the problem.

He looks at me and says, " Baby, if there's one thing for sure, it's that you and I are going to be parents. We may not know when or how, but I am committed to building our family with you."

I'm so relieved to hear his words because that's what I want as well. In the span of a year, we've experienced only one attempt and endured one heart-wrenching setback. It may not seem like much, and we're still navigating through the uncertainties, but the toll on both my body and mind has been tremendous.

MARCH 16, 2023

Once again, I managed to secure an appointment quickly for a consultation with the surgeon. "It's unusual for your fibroid to return, such occurrences are rare." he tells me. I can't help but chuckle at the irony of the situation. I also express my intention to have my fallopian tube removed. I'm a firm believer that everything happens for a reason. If there's to be surgery, let's address all potential sources of concern. Besides, removing the tube eliminates the risk of an ectopic pregnancy, a thought that brings me a measure of reassurance, shared by my partner who stands by my side

As I sign the consent forms for the operation and leave his office, a lingering phrase from a previous discussion with four doctors resurfaces in my mind, "You've got both hydrosalpinx".

Doubt gnaws at me momentarily, questioning whether I understood correctly amidst the stress and the unfamiliarity of medical jargon, expressed in English. To ease my concerns and ensure I'm on the right path, I take the proactive step of scheduling an appointment at my fertility clinic. It's a small act of self-assurance before the impending operation, a chance to confirm that I'm undertaking all necessary measures as I navigate this tumultuous journey.

MARCH 20, 2023

I take a number and sit in the waiting room. I'm desperately hoping that my intuition is mistaken. At the same time, a new discomfort on my left side has recently emerged... When my name is called, I emphasize the need to converse in French. They graciously accommodate my request, and send me back to the waiting room in the meantime. By chance, I get to see my doctor again. What a relief when she says my name and I recognize her. I already feel confident. Going through my medical file, she gets the confirmation of the previous suspicion: hydrosalpinx for both tubes. She performs another ultrasound to confirm this diagnosis. Her conclusion leaves no room for mistake; both my tubes are swollen.

— "But why? How?

— Often, when one tube is affected, the other follows. Especially with severe endometriosis like yours. I suggest removing both while you're having surgery. Right now, they're not serving any purpose anyway.

— But what if my other two embryos don't work?

— We can try again, there are many tax credits available, and at least there's a solution. It's very possible for you to conceive with IVF. You're still very young.

— Okay, but what if my fibroid comes back, or if we can't remove it completely? Am I the worst patient you've had?

— No, no, you're not the worst, don't worry. And as for your fibroid, it shouldn't come back too quickly, we'll do a transfer on a natural cycle this time, so fewer hormones.

She even appears to find all of this as wonderful news... To her, it increases the chances of success for my embryo transfer, and most importantly, I'm reassured that I won't have an ectopic pregnancy.

I'm in shock. But resilient.

I leave once again with an ultrasound of my blocked tubes and my fibroid. I have to return and sign another consent form with the surgeon and bring him these new images. I immediately called my partner and shared the news with him. He's relieved too, knowing that there's one less stressor in the equation. I feel like I haven't fully comprehended it yet; no tears have been shed, despite being informed that I'm infertile and will need IVF for life. And yet, I still have two embryos..."

Two days passed, and anxiety caught up with me, hitting me hard. Thursday evening, my partner didn't get home from work until two in the morning. Until he arrived, I spent the evening on the couch, tears streaming down my face. The pain was so intense; it felt like I was on the verge of shattering into a million pieces. I couldn't understand why my emotions hit me with such force three days after the news. Perhaps it was the realization of what lay ahead. Not only was I facing the loss of both tubes, but there was uncertainty about whether the fibroid would be completely removed. A portion of it had embedded itself deep within the uterine muscle, inaccessible without risking damage to the uterus. My thoughts fixated on the fibroid, scouring the internet for information, only to discover that I had the rarest form, known to cause miscarriages even in advanced pregnancies and interfere with embryo implantation. Nausea churned in my stomach, pain gripped me, and fear consumed me. When my partner finally arrived, my eyes were swollen from hours of crying, curled up in my pajamas with my loyal dog by my side. After enduring a major anxiety attack, despite taking medication, exhaustion finally overtook me, and I drifted into a fitful sleep in my partner's comforting embrace. For over a week, tears and a persistent knot in my stomach haunted me, reaching a crescendo one morning when I awoke with the unsettling feeling that my body and mind were on the brink of collapse, as though I might explode at any moment.

I cancelled my workday, and by some extraordinary twist of luck, I managed to see a psychologist the same day. He sensed my cry for help and luckily, my history with him from my younger days seemed to grant me some leeway. I managed to regain control gradually, but without the help of a professional, I don't think I would have gotten there as swiftly. Now, I'll be under weekly supervision. There's no denying I had reached a critical point.

APRIL 10, 2023

I've been scheduled for surgery on April 25th, and an embryo transfer is on the horizon for this summer. Though the emotional rollercoaster persists, I'm getting better at managing my anxiety. They say time has a way of healing wounds, and truer words were never spoken. I'm resolute in my decision to persist until I achieve success. I don't have any other choice anyway. Well, in reality, I do have a choice. I can choose to go on or to walk away from this journey. Ultimately, it's my body and my mind that are gearing up at the starting line, ready to tackle the marathon ahead.

I'm determined to freeze more embryos while my ovarian reserve is still favorable. I've come to terms with my decision to persevere through this journey. I count myself fortunate to live in an era where medical advancements allow miracles, and success rates are promising. As I plan a vibrant summer filled with music and cherished moments with my partner, I'm reminded of the importance of finding joy in life's simple pleasures. While my desire for children remains strong, my ultimate goal is happiness, and I refuse to endure further pain and sorrow. My therapist encourages me to embrace each day, focusing on the present moment. With two embryos still in our possession, even in the face of potential setbacks, the option of another IVF cycle remains open. I trust that my journey to parenthood will unfold in due time. Though having children later in life may not have been the path I envisioned, it has undoubtedly shaped me into a stronger, more resilient individual. I've undergone a profound transformation over the past three years. I've emerged stronger, more self-assured, and increasingly confident in myself. Through this journey, I've discovered the importance of setting boundaries and surrounding myself with supportive individuals who uplift me. I've learned to assertively say no, refusing to prioritize others' happiness over my own. My admiration for women has only deepened; I see us as resilient and remarkably strong. While my ideal scenario might have included a larger family of two or three children, I've come to accept that life doesn't always adhere to our plans. Nevertheless, the possibility of welcoming even one child into my life would be nothing short of a miracle.

Over the past year and four months, I've experienced: three months of endometriosis medication, a biopsy, an egg retrieval, three embryos, a cancelled transfer, a hysteroscopy, surgery for fibroids, a negative transfer, another cancelled transfer, and soon to come, another surgery for a fibroid and to remove my fallopian tubes. Not to mention the dozens of blood tests and vaginal ultrasounds. Only one attempt during all this time... only one!

I consider myself incredibly fortunate to have my partner by my side. I truly believe he is the most remarkable person on this planet. Not a day goes by without laughter, without affirming our love for each other and our commitment to our relationship. He often tells me, "I'd rather face life's biggest challenges with you than experience all its beautiful moments without you." There are no sweeter words a partner could say. I count my blessings daily, realizing how fortunate I am. I couldn't imagine parenthood with anyone else by my side. We're not going to give up, and I know that, if we ever run out of options, we would then consider adoption. We must not forget that we're not just infertile. We're so much more than that: human beings doing our best with a very difficult life challenge.

Living with infertility is undeniably arduous. It's normal to feel isolated, anxious about the future, to lose our bearings and question "why us?". It's not easy, but we can find our happiness. We just have to work hard and surround ourselves with the right people. I am grateful for the love in my life, for my partner, my family, my job, and my beloved dog. Each day, I strive to remember these blessings.

I understand that this journey towards parenthood involves waiting and enduring disappointments. However, I am determined to continue embracing life's vibrant colours. To do so, I prioritize my physical and mental well-being. This journey teaches us resilience and the importance of self-care. I've decided that fertility won't define me any longer. I'm committed to being healthy and enjoying life. I've accepted that I will have my children later, period. In this process, wishful thinking doesn't change the outcome. It just helps soften the time... while waiting.

We still have two precious embryos waiting in the freezer. If they don't result in a successful pregnancy, we'll embark on the journey again. As long as my body allows it, we'll persist. I hold on to the belief that someday, I will be pregnant and we will be parents.

CHAPTER 6

TO EXPLAIN THE INEXPLICABLE

By Virginie Paré

My name is Virginie, and I'm 33 years old. I'm a chiropractor, blessed to share my life with the man I've loved for a decade now. Our story began through mutual friends. Initially, our relationship was purely platonic, but deep down, I had a feeling he was meant for me. I vividly remember writing down this intuition in my journal at the time, and today, I take great pleasure in reminding Jean-François whenever he occasionally doubts that same intuition. A few months into our acquaintance, supported by a few alcoholic beverages for courage, I mustered up the courage to take the first steps toward the next chapter of our lives. It happened in the dimly lit basement of a bar on St-Denis Street, in Montreal. Our journey together was marked by numerous travels, the onset of my chiropractic career, sharing our first apartment in the Plateau, countless moments of laughter, evenings spent with friends, and an abundance of joy. During those early days, I often found myself the target of remarks and inquiries from friends, wondering when the baby plans would overshadow our many escapades. They cautioned against waiting too long, citing the uncertainty of what the future might hold.

The desire to become a mother has always been present within me. To be honest, at first, I wasn't sure if this desire stemmed from societal expectations subtly instilled in us or if it was truly my own. A few years after graduating as a chiropractor, my best friend Anne surprised me by arranging a postgraduate course in perinatal chiropractic care and had already enrolled me. Thanks to her bold gesture of friendship, I spent three wonderful years honing my skills, learning how to provide the best care for expectant mothers and newborns. During those same three years, I also joined the team at an alternative medicine center focused on perinatal care, in addition to flourishing in a wonderful clinic where I had become a co-owner. It is safe to say that I came across pregnant bellies by the dozen and I felt exactly like where I belonged. Being surrounded by young families in my professional environment helped crystallize that previously ambiguous desire, to the point where I often joked that my ovaries were starting to itch. For Jean-François, the desire to start a family was certainly present, but we both wanted to fully experience our life as a couple before embarking on this beautiful journey. So, we waited until the eve of our thirtieth birthday to plan our ideal vision board for the next chapter of our family life:

Our first pregnancy was meant to unfold in the comfort of our condo in Villeray. We dreamed of becoming parents in the heart of Montreal, relishing in the delights of neighborhood life. Picture-perfect walks with the stroller to Jean-Talon market, sipping iced coffees, before ending up at the Jarry park for an afternoon treat. Naturally, we envisioned welcoming our bundle of joy during the warmth of summer. Just before the desire for baby #2 arose, we would begin our search for a long-term residence on the North Shore of the island, where both of us had grown up. The goal was to find a multi-generational home that would allow my parents to move in with us. This way, we could continue expanding our family with two or even three pregnancies... Dog, inground pool, the whole shebang.

I was living in a fantasy world of glittery unicorns, where the little pink lines appeared as swiftly and effortlessly as a Monday morning.

Anxiety crept into our intimacy swiftly and insidiously. As early as the second month of trying, plagued by relentless and destructive questioning about my fertile crescent, I found myself tumbling prematurely into the endless spiral of unattainable surrender. The ability to let go, often cited as the number one obstacle for any woman facing infertility. My body possessed all the necessary ingredients to reach this miraculous physiological transformation that led to conception, so what was going wrong? With my performance anxiety taking the reins, there was no way I would passively wait for months to pass by, and remain inactive—I wanted to take action, right then and there. My first instinct was to turn to alternative medicines: chiropractic care, acupuncture, naturopathy, nutrition, and even some evidence-lacking trials that provided me with solace and peace of mind. In my mind, I approached this with a simple medical history that perhaps required just a few tweaks here and there:

A 30-year-old woman, nulliparous (a term used to identify a woman who has never been pregnant, which, among my top 5 most disliked words, ranks quite high—I find it derogatory even though it has done me no harm), active, non-smoker, socially drinks alcohol, avoids drugs, takes no medications, no known health history, except perhaps a slightly fragile digestive system, regular menstrual cycle, able to recognize signs of ovulation always around the fourteenth day of the month, has discontinued the use of female contraceptives for the past 5 years, etc. For several months, and still to this day, I have been working on my lifestyle habits to maximize my chances of conceiving naturally. Natural products, meditation, rituals, gratitude, therapies, stress management, an exemplary diet based on my hormonal cycle, and so forth. Though my belly hasn't yet swelled with pregnancy, these changes have brought me immense well-being and, most importantly, made me aware of the ironic lack of knowledge I had about women's health.

My sister and I are the joyful miracle of a delightful cliché of parents who, forty years ago now, met in an emergency room, where they both were beginning their careers, my father as a doctor and my mother as a nurse. Our parents were invaluable allies in our fertility journey. Sometimes they'd explain the tests we had to undergo in greater detail, knowing the doctors or nurses we would encounter, confirming the changes we felt with certain medications, but most importantly, they provided empathy and comfort from the very beginning. Jean-François and I never hid our challenges in conceiving from our family members, colleagues, or friends. For us, this decision was incredibly liberating. It allowed us, to some extent, to feel less alone and especially to realize how fortunate we were to be so well supported. A few months into our natural attempts, I had a conversation with my mother over a glass of her favorite Chardonnay. I asked her if she remembered how long it took for her to see a positive test result. After a moment of reflection, she admitted to trying for a few months and then stopping since it was clear it wasn't working. I asked her if she thought about it a lot, if her desire generated intrusive thoughts like I was beginning to notice in myself. Her response was the singular memory of being shocked by her best friend's pregnancy announcement, but nothing more. Her positive test followed that announcement two months later. I remember deducing that the creeping distress I was gradually feeling might possibly become a distant memory in thirty years.

Unfortunately, the months passed by with a disheartening sameness. As the critical twenty-eighth day of my cycle approached, I would often call Anne in a bit of a panic because I felt no signs of early pregnancy. Her pep talk, worthy of a professional cheerleader, had less and less effect on the emptiness that was gradually growing, both subjectively and objectively, in my belly. We had reached the six-month mark of natural attempts. We were still within the normal timeframe, but my anxiety would occasionally poison my thoughts. Jean-François remained optimistic, comforting me with each arrival of my menstrual cycle. After several discussions, we decided to make an appointment with my family doctor for advice. Despite not being alarmed by our situation due to our health profiles, my doctor still prescribed the necessary fertility tests: blood tests, pelvic ultrasound, hysterosalpingography, and a sperm analysis for Jean-François. She also talked to us about the various fertility clinics available for further steps. At that moment, my ego was dealt a heavy blow. Virginie Paré, a proponent of vitalism, needing medicine, drugs, interventions to help me achieve a physiological cascade of events that my body knows perfectly well how to orchestrate itself? It was, at that moment, impossible for me to accept.

11:11, make a wish: I wish to become a mother.

The months that followed were still challenging for Jean-François and me. We experienced our first losses related to our picture-perfect vision of the family chapter. In the midst of a pandemic, we decided it was wise to sell our condo and unfortunately, remove the possibility of a pregnancy on the island from our vision board. The pandemic brought its share of destabilizing events for our relationship in regards to our professional activities. Like many families in Quebec, we found ourselves spending a lot of time together, and we were lucky to fully appreciate every moment. Several times, I was told to appreciate the silence and calm in my home because many of our friends were facing a completely different reality. It was a heartbreaking comment, as I increasingly dreamed of chaos, cries, and messiness, yet I overflowed with empathy for those who longed to trade places with us, even for just a moment. We also experienced a halt in our efforts to find the cause of our fertility challenges. This imposed pause was reassuring to me because we needed time to continue our natural process. The impatient side of me would have struggled to allow this break otherwise, feeling like we were losing precious months. Slowly, I entertained the idea of perhaps consulting a fertility clinic, just to explore our options. However, the infamous biological clock rang loudly within me, like Captain Hook's watch inside the belly of the crocodile. Tick, tock, tick, tock.

I continued my appointments with my various holistic therapists, whom I affectionately called my "fertility army." When our lives gradually returned to some semblance of normalcy, my naturopath asked me if I was giving myself space to have a child. I pondered this question deeply. I was working a lot, long physically demanding hours, had little time to rest, my personal schedule was planned to the minute, leaving me very little time... to just be. The idea of slowing down at work was very anxiety-inducing for me. It was inconceivable for me to consider dropping patients for fear of being seen as lazy. With the help of my partner, I was able to recognize the irrationality behind this destructive thought and that it might be preferable to reduce my workload to maximize our chances, especially if we were to start fertility treatments at a clinic. And so, I had to ask the owner of the perinatal clinic where I worked for a "fertility leave." This kind and understanding soul made this experience, which was so heart-wrenching for me, easy and obvious to take. A few months later, I bid farewell to wonderful colleagues and patients for what I thought would be a short period of time, just enough to get pregnant and get through the first trimester. Life had other plans.

Blood tests, imaging, and sperm analysis later, no issues were detected. We were even sold a bit of a dream during the hysterosalpingography, with the hope that many women became pregnant after this procedure. The test involved injecting contrast liquid into the uterus and fallopian tubes to discover any abnormalities. For me, everything looked perfect. So, I received a free and painless "cleanup" of my female labyrinth. The state of fragility and vulnerability I was in led to a higher disappointment when I realized that the so-called positive outcomes of a test or miraculous technique were not at all beneficial for us. The summer of 2020 marked the beginning of our journey at the fertility clinic. Several discussions with Jean-François and some of my closest friends helped me realize that ultimately, what I desired most in the world was to hold our baby in my arms, and I could allow myself a helping hand to achieve that. Still, I felt an internal duality in accepting medical assistance that might eventually lead to taking medications or even surgical interventions when, to date, no problems had been identified. The start of our journey at the clinic also marked the imaginary barrier I had to overcome in accepting that we were now indeed talking about infertility, a term that was difficult for me to accept. During our first phone call with our fertility doctor, he summarized our situation as follows:

— "Essentially, your partner's sperm just needs a little assistance finding its way through your plumbing. We'll try a few inseminations, and by December, you should be pregnant.

Perhaps for some, this humor-infused presentation could have been reassuring. For me, I found it insulting. Why not talk about the real issues? I desperately needed explanations, a reason to help me make sense of it all. With my numerous questions, I eventually understood that the cause of infertility remained unexplained, that both my partner's and my own results were all fine and normal. Endometriosis could have been a consideration, but since I didn't fit the clinical picture, further investigation wasn't necessary. Besides, "pregnancy was the treatment for endometriosis," the doctor confirmed.

Blow out the thirty-first candle, make a wish: I want to become a mother.

"Inexplicable": suggests something that cannot be explained, implies lack of rational reason. The uncertainty, once again. What wasn't working in me, or in us, no one knew. I was told to be patient, encouraged with reassurances that it could still happen naturally or that it would happen eventually. But no one knew for sure.

Nonetheless, we waited until the beginning of 2021 to start the inseminations. I still needed time, and we were in the process of buying a house. We found THE multi-generational house of our dreams that met all our criteria. During our first visit, I remember experiencing a moment of panic while touring the rooms on the second floor: What if we were never able to fill them? Jean-François, always reassuring in his words, comforted me by saying that we were getting a little closer each day to realizing our dream and that, on the contrary, perhaps these beautiful empty rooms would send a positive message to the universe... He knew my "love language." I thought to myself that we had envisioned a messy version of our family chapter and that we were still slowly making it happen.

In January 2021, on the first day of my cycle, I started taking tablets that would stimulate the growth of one or more ovarian follicles. Just one medication to maximize our chances—it was acceptable, not the end of the world, I could do it. At the ultrasound on day 12 of the cycle, the same gynecologist (Ascendant: plumber) confirmed the presence of two follicles and exclaimed loudly, "Twins!!!" I had mixed feelings about his reaction. I understood statistically that our chances were higher for twins with the presence of two little follicles, but could we really shout it from the rooftops already? Nevertheless, we decided to ride the wave of this good news and be excited about the possibility of having our hands doubly full in nine months. The procedure would take place a few days later. All I had to do was inject a medication that would trigger ovulation thirty-six hours before the insemination. I managed my first injection. I had given myself enough time to go through the mental process that led me to accept the medical assistance and, most importantly, to be grateful for the scientific advancements that might allow Jean-François and me to become parents. As I picked up my prescription at the pharmacy the same day, I crossed paths with a woman picking up medication for what seemed to me like in vitro fertilization. The mountain of boxes and containers of medication literally triggered significant anxiety in me, with nausea and cold sweats. I remembered thanking some unknown force for not being in a situation where in vitro fertilization was THE answer to our needs. With a lot of arrogance, I mentioned to Jean-François that it was impossible for me to even consider that we might need to resort to this alternative. The mental journey was not quite complete after all. The infamous injection still went well, as I was fortunate to have it supervised by a nurse with forty years of experience—my mom—who made sure that our clumsy hands didn't contaminate the needle by accidentally dropping it on the counter. As the injection was an inherent part of the process, I found it important to ask Jean-François for permission to invite my mother into this new kind of intimacy. My brain had some difficulty retaining all the information from the quick crash course on "how to inject" that the fertility clinic nurse had delivered at a much faster pace than the nursing techniques in college.

Sitting uncomfortably on the table, waiting for the doctor, my emotions fluctuated between excitement and pessimism. I struggled to understand what this technique would offer us beyond what we were already capable of doing in the comfort of our intimacy. Excellent quality of sperm sample, an intervention that literally lasted forty-five seconds, a knowing look between Jean-François and me that said it all about the speed of it... So, we left for home with a lingering feeling of absurdity in the back of our throats. The few days that followed were marked by nausea and overwhelming fatigue. Excitement and anticipation filled us throughout the painful two weeks separating the insemination from the pregnancy test. I waited until the recommended day to purchase the pregnancy test because the urge to do it earlier would have been too intense. At the pharmacy, I even bought a lottery ticket ironically to symbolize the chance that might finally be on our side. It was Jean-François who looked at the test result and gently informed me that I was not pregnant. My eyes were filled with questions. What had happened? Why all these symptoms? Was I being excessive with this desire to the point of imagining physical manifestations? Was I going crazy? I was more traumatized by my body's reaction following the intervention than by the negative test. Crouched in a small ball in my bathtub, I called my best friend in tears, hysterical, on the verge of hyperventilation.

"Vie (it's my nickname), talk to me, what's going on? I don't understand, breathe slowly with me..." As I slowly regained my composure and my normal breath, we hypothesized that my body's reaction to the hormones ingested before the procedure was normal. So, I wasn't crazy, my symptoms were real, but they weren't related to pregnancy. My clinician's ego took a good hit in the face. Why hadn't I thought of that?

I was in my office at the clinic, with five days left to wait before taking the pregnancy test following the second insemination. I found it difficult to concentrate; I couldn't stop thinking about it. I was in a state of hypervigilance, analyzing every twinge or heaviness I dared to perceive. I hated seeing myself like this. How could I let intrusive thoughts hold so much importance, making this experience so unpleasant? That's what I voiced to my psychologist during our weekly appointment.

"With everything you've told me, I believe it would be appropriate to consider introducing an antidepressant to help you," she said.

The effect of a hara-kiri on my cognition. I am acutely aware that I have been living with a high level of anxiety for several years, but it has been manageable. I have a fear of giving too much space to this anxiety that would lead me to no longer appreciate life as I have always savored it. A few years ago, I made the most beautiful promise to myself by ensuring to prevent any signs leading to possible depression. I decided that psychotherapy would always be a preferred ally to maintain an acceptable mental health. I had been seeing this psychologist for several months. I was adamant from the beginning of our journey about my motivation towards any alternative that would spare me the tumultuous path that depression could lead to, especially the medication associated with it. This sentence shattered the trust I had in my therapist. Insulted, disillusioned, worried, I rushed to my dear neighbors. My pale and lifeless face immediately alarmed my mother. Between sobs, I asked my parents if they perceived any signs of depression in me and if, in their opinion, I should consider taking medication. My father, who since March 2020 had been saddened by prescribing this type of medication too often, was dismayed to see me shattered by this recommendation and also doubted the relevance of this help for me, especially in the context of fertility. Spouse, friends, colleagues, parents, all heard my heartfelt plea, begging them to be honest with me and indicate if, from their point of view, I was dangerously veering towards the dark side. Although all shared my father's opinion, I realized in that instant that I was walking on very thin ice, putting my mental health to a severe test. I had confidence in my abilities and my toolbox to continue this journey without medication, but I vowed to be cautious for the steps that were yet to come.

It was the day of the second pregnancy test. I hadn't even bothered to get one because I knew my period was imminent. Jean-François was finishing up renovations for the shared laundry room we had envisioned. For ecological reasons, we found it responsible to have a single space in the basement for both units. I had also imagined a pleasant and well-thought-out area that would make our lives easier, knowing it was a frequently used room when the family expanded. Jean-François's best friend had just adopted a puppy, Wesley, and was bombarding us with photos, knowing I was a huge fan of dogs, unlike Jean-François. The night before, we had even received a video that comforted me, as I had just learned that a very close friend was pregnant. She had the delicacy to announce it to me over the phone and gave me time to digest the news at my own pace. Upon receiving the video, Jean-François candidly suggested we consider getting a small dog in about six months if our situation hadn't changed. Words failed me to express the gratitude I felt for being able to share my life with this man. Behind this proposition was a reasoning whose ultimate goal was to bring me a little sweetness and lightness in this storm of emotions and turmoil. Between installing clotheslines and watching little Wesley's antics, our friends wrote to us that there was still a puppy available at the breeder's, in case we were interested. Not at all intrigued by this proposition, already feeling lucky that Jean-François was considering the idea of a dog in six months, I replied that it was just postponed. I looked up from my phone to meet Jean-François's thoughtful and serious gaze.

— "It could still be a good idea to experience this adventure together with our friends.

— My love, are you serious? Getting a dog is really not a small decision to make... And we're not prepared at all."

He then asked me to call the breeder for information. The last little eight-week-old border collie was already reserved, but since the lady really liked our friends, she preferred to let us have him. We had twenty-four hours to pick him up. In fifteen minutes, everything was settled. I tossed my credit card to my parents and asked them to buy everything I needed to welcome a puppy. I was screaming, jumping, and crying tears of joy. So, on a Sunday afternoon, we raced to Megantic to pick up our little Moose, slightly exceeding the limits of the curfew still in effect at that time. Sorry, Mr. Prime Minister, it was a case of force majeure for the sake of improving someone's mental health.

If some find the phenomenon of "dog mom" excessive, you can imagine the transition to a "dog mom", when dealing with infertility. Nevertheless, Moose's arrival brought a sense of lightness to the house that was greatly appreciated. My thoughts were now focused on him, almost forgetting the necessary steps for the third and final insemination. It wasn't the failure that destabilized us this time, but rather the waiting period we had to endure before taking action for the next steps. Personally, I had to slowly start a mental process to accept and embrace what was shaping up to be the next stage: in vitro fertilization.

Before the steps that led us to the in vitro fertilization process, I never felt fully committed to this assisted reproduction journey. I played the hypocrite by reminding myself that our diagnosis, if it was indeed one, did not exclude the possibility of natural pregnancy. However, due to lack of patience, I still decided to explore our various options. I also realized that I had no friends or family members who had reached this stage and therefore no one to answer my questions and concerns.

The process began in August 2021. The ultrasounds, blood tests, and injections went smoothly. I was fortunate to go through this process during a summer vacation period, which gave me more flexibility at work to cancel and reschedule my patients' appointments, allowing me ample time for my own follow-ups. During the injection period, Jean-François worked nights, so I often found myself alone, improvising as a "chemist-junky." With two or three injections, sometimes painless but occasionally feeling like a thin stream of peri-umbilical lava, the progression of my follicular production went quite well. The days leading up to the egg retrieval quickly became unbearable. I felt like I was incubating dragon eggs, with the ever-present heaviness in my abdomen, not to mention the hormonal side effects. I anticipated the night before the embryo transfer to be the most difficult, not knowing what to expect and considering the complexity of the procedure. So, I took the day before the transfer to do things I particularly enjoy, to offer myself some comfort and pleasure, as well as to reduce anxiety as much as possible: walking in the forest with my dog, reading, taking a bubble bath, and finally, cooking what I craved: corn dogs. Understand that this craving was really out of the ordinary considering my diet guided by my hormonal cycle. No, corn dogs did not fit the recommendations for the ovulatory phase. We showed up on a rainy Saturday morning for our appointment to retrieve the precious treasure I had been incubating for two weeks. A total of 19 follicles were retrieved, ten eggs were mature, and 6 champions had successfully undergone fertilization. These were the results the embryologist revealed to us the next morning, promptly at seven o'clock. We were warned to expect to lose a few more blastocysts before embryo freezing. Since I had quite high hormone levels, it was safer to avoid a fresh embryo transfer, so in the end, we ended up with four excellent-quality little popsicles. The week following the egg retrieval is possibly the moment in this whole process where women display an inexplicable mental strength. Not only do we have to navigate the hormone drop, but we also have to live with the idea that a part of us is evolving in a laboratory far from our warm uterus, all while waiting for news from the embryologist who will announce how many embryos have survived 24 hours-three-days-five- days later.

The day before the first transfer, the embryologist confirmed our appointment time and reminded me not to forget to arrive with a full bladder. I took this request very seriously, thinking there was a very high correlation between the success of the transfer and the fullness of my bladder. I was lying in the procedure room with the ultrasound probe on my abdomen when the nurse exclaimed that my bladder was far too full and that I needed to empty it by twenty milliliters to provide a better view of my uterus. I had to summon superhuman effort from my pelvic floor to resist the urgent need to empty my bladder completely. By the third attempt, tears welled up in my eyes, and I felt pain radiating into my back as my bladder cried out for relief. I felt ridiculous for letting my perfectionism take over in this absurd task where I could have simply ingested a normal amount of liquid and let nature take its course. After the procedure, the staff placed me on a stretcher and asked me to stay there for a few minutes without further explanation. Thinking it was to maximize the chances of our little embryo attaching by defying gravity, as was the case during inseminations, I had to wait what felt like an eternity before I could finally urinate. I was asked to lie down for ten minutes, which I was unable to do. Quite alarmed by the situation, as I was afraid of jeopardizing our chances, a nurse finally reassured me that the situation would likely have no impact on the process. Additionally, she advised me that eventually (since it would be the same recommendations during pregnancy ultrasounds), I could simply empty my bladder an hour before the procedure and start hydrating once in the waiting room. Too little, too late.

We received the call for our result on a Monday, late morning. It was November 1st, a beautiful windy but sunny autumn day. I was outside with Jean-François and my dog, practicing his frisbee catches. I had trouble putting my phone back in my pocket for fear of missing the call. A feeling of serenity enveloped me; I was just fine, and I didn't want to think about what my life would be like in a few minutes.

When the nurse said my name, I knew it was negative. I even felt like telling her she didn't need to continue. I wanted to spare her the discomfort of having to tell a hopeful couple that it wouldn't be this time. I also wanted to spare myself what feels like a stab to the soul. I've never bungee jumped in my life, but I'm convinced that the sensation I felt when I heard the compassionate voice announcing my result is the same as the split second before leaping into the void, an endless void for me. I had trouble looking at Jean-François. Seeing the disappointment on his face would just make it all feel even more real.

— "I don't understand; you're so young."

That's what the nurse told me afterward. Second blow to the heart. I didn't understand either. I would have loved to understand. Was anyone, anywhere, understanding what was happening? An intervention that guaranteed us a success rate between 50% and 60% and still nothing. What wasn't working with me?

The intensity level was so high after the announcement that instead of allowing myself to fully experience my emotions, my nervous system decided to simply shut down. After a few minutes of intense crying, I was overcome by a massive wave of fatigue that led me to sleep for the rest of the day. This avoidance mechanism orchestrated by some part of me clearly didn't consider the extreme disappointment the first split second before waking up. The moment you realize it definitely wasn't a dream and you plunge even deeper into the emotional distress that an HCG level of 0 can leave you in. Before the call ended, I had managed to utter a complete sentence amid three or four sobs.

— "What's next?"

"You stop your medication, wait for your period, and then you can call us to schedule the second transfer."

The end of that painful call.

The waiting is possibly the most draining aspect of my fertility journey. The four-to-six-month delay before seeing my doctor again, the postponement of my transfer by a month, a new test to take, and nothing to do but wait for the call to schedule the appointment, being on a waiting list... It may seem trivial, but for me, it had the effect of draining my optimism. The helplessness associated with this waiting is a loss of control that my organizational rigidity struggled to handle. In June 2021, I began the process for ovarian stimulation in preparation for my first IVF. Injections every day, side effects every hour, but intoxicated with an incomparable lightness of heart, we were getting closer to our dream. During the first follow-up ultrasound for follicular growth, in a dimly lit office with air conditioning struggling to mask the early summer heat, the doctor, who didn't seem to be having the best of days, abruptly asked me the reason for my infertility.

— "Unexplained.

"We're going to stop all this; you're not responding enough to the medications. I only see four follicles, and that's not normal for someone with your profile."

I had considered several scenarios for this meeting. Never had this possibility crossed my imagination. From the beginning, I was made to feel like an "easy" case. The tests were good, I was young and in good health. What wasn't working with me? Letting my emotions out in public isn't easy for me. Not out of pride, but because I don't want to make people around me uncomfortable. Don't worry, I understand the psychological issue behind this behavior, and I'm working on it. After the brief exchange with the doctor, I collapsed in the nurse's office, who told me I had to wait another two months before restarting the process. Wait... again! This turn of events made me feel like the caricature of the donkey with a carrot tied in front of its nose, allowing it to move forward. We were so close to our dream, but an inexplicable force still prevented us from getting there. It was frustrating. Those two months seemed so insignificant, but after two years of waiting, no matter how much I worked on my resilience and patience, I allowed myself to feel overwhelmed at that moment.

When the nurse confirmed that the second transfer could take place at the beginning of my next hormonal cycle, we were literally stunned. We had never encountered such speed in a sequence of events before. For once, we didn't have to wait; we could continue right there, right now, a small whiff of beta-carotene.

My first frozen embryo transfer was conducted under a substituted cycle, meaning with a good dose of hormones before, during, and after the transfer. I asked myself many questions to determine if it wasn't too much to ask of my body to go through all these steps again in such a short period. I had a few days left to make my final decision. Always torn between my desire, which would lead me to exceed my bodily capacities, and, on the other hand, my wisdom and reasoning, that's when a moment of clarity crossed my mind. Why not return to immerse myself in my love-hate relationship with support groups on social media? I had been maintaining this relationship with them for several months, with intermittent breaks of no more than forty-eight hours due to overwhelming anxiety after reading the testimonials. "Sign up, unsubscribe": that was my mantra.

But perhaps this time, it could be useful to me... I really wanted to find out if someone shared the same story and if, faced with a decision like the one we had to make, happy endings had occurred.

Rewriting my post about ten times, I was a bit afraid to share my story for the first time, especially on this type of platform. Jean-François looked at me with a lot of apprehension. He knew he might have to intervene in the coming days with his comforting and optimistic speech to calm my alarmist scenarios after reading heartbreaking testimonies.

A few hours after "my big public outing," I was contacted by Sophie, a young mother who, after her second transfer, finally had her little miracle. It was the first time I had exchanged with someone who could understand what I was going through. I was so grateful for her sharing her story, her encouragement, and her advice. They confirmed my desire to move forward with the second transfer. I immediately withdrew from the group for the umpteenth time, finally finding the comfort I was looking for in this fellow IVF warrior.

As a chiropractor, I am fortunate to exchange daily with many wonderful humans who all have an impact on my professional life, and sometimes even my personal life. The famous question, which many women in a similar situation probably greet with a lot of bitterness, was regularly asked to me:

— "Do you have any children?

— No, not yet.

Five years ago, this question was trivial for me. Today, it has a tightening effect on my heart. On days when I give more space to my anger and rage, I question the relevance of this question. On the other hand, having a practice focused on perinatology, I find it normal that some of my patients are interested in knowing if my empathy comes from personal experience or if I simply perfected my listening skills.

Between my two frozen embryo transfers, I was asked this question by a patient. I must admit that I was still digesting the recent failure very badly. For some reason, I didn't feel like continuing with my usual pre-chewed response. So, I replied that we were currently in an in vitro fertilization process. A soft light then crossed her eyes as she confided in me that she had undergone this process for her son. This patient then shared with me that, following a first failed transfer, she had decided, for her second one, to take a break from work between the day of the procedure and her blood test. She focused on her well-being and especially did a variety of things that made her feel good.

Her second transfer was a success. She highly recommended that I do the same.

Normally, I don't pay much attention to unsolicited advice. It's just sometimes overwhelming to be constantly targeted with information that, mostly, is just a collection of thin evidence. On several occasions, I had to use my acting skills to show interest in these famous pieces of advice coming from people who often aren't even close to experiencing a fraction of what we're going through. I'll always remember a conversation with a clerk at a natural products store who, after guessing that the supplements in my order were for fertility purposes, candidly told me to stop smoking weed. Looking back, what frustrates me about this situation is that I didn't stand up for myself and instead thanked him for his "valuable" advice. Oh, but I still fantasize to this day about the raw speech I would have liked to give him. However, I discussed this idea with Jean-François (the idea of taking time off work, not quitting smoking weed since I never really started...) and we agreed that a small dose of rest, mixed with plenty of endorphins could help us stack the odds in our favor. For once, I considered this advice to be valuable.

It was November 23, 2021, a thin blanket of snow covered the ground, but not so much as to stress us out, excited to hit the road in the midst of traffic, heading to our second embryo transfer. I was beyond excited, at the peak of happiness. We were getting closer to our miracle, and Christmas was just around the corner.

I'm not one to find Christmas a painful time, even for the past four years of trying to expand our family. However, I avoid self-sabotage by disappearing completely from social media between December 23 and January 15 to avoid stumbling upon pregnancy announcements. Nonetheless, the frenzy surrounding this period nourishes my soul greatly and does wonders for my inner child. I was on the stretcher before entering the operating room. Jean-François and I were looking at a travel guide, planning our getaway intended to take our minds off the endless wait post-transfer. I longed to see New York with its Christmas decorations, a desire I'd cherished for a long time.

The second transfer unfolded in calmness, love, and comfort. Both of us left with our small dark photo illuminated by a thin white line that gave us all the hope in the world.

I woke up forty-eight hours after the transfer with blood on my underwear. I was petrified. I remembered having a similar discharge during the first transfer just before the blood test. So, I was convinced we would face another failure. Nevertheless, I decided to call the nurses' emergency line. I was in tears, struggling to breathe, speak, and explain my distress. With reassuring words like "Calm down, ma'am," the nurse tried to explain that it didn't mean anything and that stress wasn't good for me or the baby. If you don't want to receive a piercing gaze, a sharp retort, or perhaps even a physical manifestation of increased rage, know that every woman undergoing fertility treatment knows that stress isn't good for her, and no, it's not possible to stop thinking about it. We think about it differently as the years go by. Instead, try something like, "I hear what you're saying; it must not be easy."

The beginning of our stay in the Big Apple was marked by my frequent stops to the restroom to check if there were still traces of blood and the compassionate looks from my beloved, who would ask me, "How is it?" after each of my trips. On November 30, 2021, I woke up, but this time, I had vaginal bleeding that was nothing like what I had been experiencing for the past five days. I was used to following the recommendations given to me since the beginning of this process, but that morning, I decided to disobey. I took a urine pregnancy test. It wasn't my first rodeo. Over the past two years, I had taken a few, and I had also tried to hallucinate the two parallel lines several times. But this time, I wasn't hallucinating. I could clearly see two beautiful parallel lines. I emerged from the bathroom with the pregnancy test in hand, and I could see that Jean-François was ready to deliver his "post-pee test speech," which he had given so many times to lift my spirits. He didn't have time to speak before I told him it was positive. We looked at each other silently for a few seconds, astonished, astounded. He cautiously suggested that the bleeding might be due to the hormones I was taking, as the nurse had reminded us several times.

I had to grieve the pregnancy announcements as seen in movies or, in fact, as experienced by a good majority of couples around me. Surprising Jean-François with the coveted little +1, the hallmark moment of many relationships, seemed light-years away from our reality. When we finally got our positive result, both of us doubted, and we agreed to wait for the blood test a few days later. However, the fifteen other positive urine tests (yes, fifteen) and my strange food aversions were starting to ring a bell. Finally, as my intuition or those fifteen tests confirmed, we received the long-awaited call with the positive result.

I wish I could tell you that this is the end...

A few weeks after confirming the test, I experienced bleeding again. I had to undergo another blood test with a follow-up forty-eight hours later. It was December 21st, just three days before the Christmas holidays. My schedule was quite busy, and there was no room for any obstacle to disrupt this pre-holiday ministerial agenda.

My phone rang between two patient appointments—it was the nurse from the medical clinic where I was being monitored for my pregnancy.

— "Virginie, your hormone levels have only increased by forty units when they should have doubled or tripled. It looks very bleak, it's probably over."

"I was frozen, unable to speak. All I could do was wait for nature to take its course and start the process that would slowly kill my dream. With some unknown strength, I managed to treat the few remaining patients with alarming focus and a smile far from reassuring. The journey back home was filled with my screams, attempting to release a fraction of my pain. When I reached Jean-François, we both collapsed on the floor, crying over the misfortune that struck us once again.

The next day, after what I would describe as the worst night of my life, I had to gather my courage and care for my patients. I was still experiencing a high level of emotional distress and needed someone to help me put things into perspective and find a parcel of courage that would help me move forward. After a precious call with Anne, who was just as devastated as I was and couldn't understand the "wait and see" approach proposed to me after the obvious miscarriage, Jean-François and I decided to go to the gynecological emergency room to turn the page on this brief and painful chapter. At triage, the nurse confirmed to me, without compassion, that we should not expect a different outcome and that things looked very bad for the future. We were placed in a cubicle where we occasionally had visits from doctors or nurses to explain how the next few hours would unfold. They had to confirm the outcome of the situation with an ultrasound before proceeding with any other procedures."

During the in vitro fertilization process and the subsequent transfers, we have to undergo several ultrasounds to confirm various values: presence and growth of follicles, presence of cysts, thickness of the endometrium, etc. The majority of these ultrasounds are done transvaginally. To this day, I've lost count of how many times I've had to sit my bare bottom as close as possible to the void with my feet in the stirrups, my hips rolled inward, to allow me the maximum amount of modesty that this vulnerable position can offer. Sometimes, when we're lucky, the gel covering the probe is at room temperature, sparing us the icy surprise at the start of the exam. So, I prepared in the same way for the ultrasound that would confirm the outcome of our nightmare. I struggle to describe the radiologist's astonishment when he entered the room and did not expect to see his next patient undressed like that. This ridiculous situation allowed me to hear a small laugh from Jean-François, and despite my discomfort, the absurdity of the situation felt like a thin ray of warmth amidst the storm of sadness that had been looming over our heads for the past twenty-four hours.

— "So, what do we have here? Excellent, I can see it here, and here. Beautiful heart, everything looks good.

— WHAT? I've just been told I was having a miscarriage. I don't understand, it's impossible.

— Look, I'm not sure what to tell you, all I see here is a beautiful baby, with a heart.

I turned to Jean-François, who at the same moment burst into tears. Tears of relief, of happiness, of incomprehension. We could only extract very few answers from our multiple questions to the doctor who met with us after the ultrasound. The hypothesis of the lost twin crept into the conversation, accompanied by a brief explanation regarding the specificity of imaging compared to blood tests. So, we could return home, relieved, and continue our journey without too many worries...

If only!

During my first prenatal appointment, our doctor unfortunately informed us that she found our fetus to be very underdeveloped for ten weeks. So, we had to wait seven agonizing days to check its growth. Perhaps, by then, nature would take care of the situation. Yet another déjà vu feeling. My father was waiting for us in the office next door, and I managed to hold back my tears for a maximum of five steps. Jean-François briefly explained the situation to him, asking the same questions we had asked our doctor thirty seconds earlier, but we were so shaken that we constantly needed reassurance. We were searching for an encouraging answer. My father, who had set aside his obstetric practice since the early 2000s, gave us the same answers, repeatedly, phrased differently, but still nothing to reassure us. We just had to be patient.

Another endless and painful wait to endure.

I was alone in the clinic waiting room. Due to COVID-19, partners were not allowed during prenatal appointments.

Knowing the possible outcomes of the appointment, my doctor kindly agreed to see me at the end of her day, allowing Jean-François to wait in my father's office and join us once the clinic was empty. It was a huge privilege, and I was aware and grateful for it. "Haters are gonna hate," but at that point, if that's all I had left? I'm convinced I was on the brink of a panic attack, sandwiched between the outdated editions of conventional women's magazines, placed on each side of my uncomfortable chair in the waiting room. I tried everything to calm myself: meditation, deep breathing, videos, and photos of Moose. My stress level was similar to that of a CEO in the midst of an economic crisis.

— "The heart is there, and... yes, it looks like it has indeed grown well."

I burst into tears. The convulsions of my abdomen made it impossible for my doctor to continue the examination. Finally seeing the little parallel bars on my pregnancy test, I thought the roller coaster of emotions was behind us. Clearly, I had gone from the kiddie roller coaster to the Monster roller coaster from our local amusement park. My doctor released us in a much lighter atmosphere than when I arrived, with the hope of seeing us again in a month.

A week later, we went for our nuchal translucency scan. We had rescheduled the appointment because Jean-François was leaving for warmer climates with his family to celebrate his father's sixtieth birthday. I had decided not to join the celebrations for obvious reasons. I woke up with a strange wave of anxiety, an odd intuition, yet I tried to convince myself to be happy because today, I would see our baby. My friend Julie, who worked at the clinic where the examination was taking place, invited us to wait in her office. She and Jean-François were talking about his last trip with great passion, but on my side, things were not going well at all. I was probably experiencing PTSD from my recent medical appointments. Julie sensed my catastrophic energy and discreetly tried to distract me. We were invited into a dark room with the imaging technician. From the beginning of the examination, she struggled to find our little one. As she adjusted some settings, she explained that the different colored lines on the screen were the blood vessels of my uterus, and our fetus should be there, but all that was visible on the screen was a black spot. My body tensed up, and my defense mechanisms kicked in immediately. I wanted to flee, to leave the clinic, to start running. I was short of breath. The technician burst into tears. Jean-François didn't understand; he had so many questions, but I was simply unable to answer him. I heard a continuous loud buzzing that confused my brain; I just wanted to leave. It was over.

I had to wait six days before my appointment for a dilation and curettage (D&C). That was the chosen path to analyze the genetic background of the embryo and hopefully get some answers to our many questions. I was a human grave for six days. I have trouble recalling the period between the miscarriage announcement and the D&C. I had to take several days off from work because I couldn't concentrate anymore. Contrary to what social judgment recommends, I didn't wait three months to announce it to our relatives. It was hard to hide, especially since many people knew about the transfer in early December, and I needed my friends during the struggles encountered in the first weeks of pregnancy. I will never regret my early announcement because the support from our friends, colleagues, and parents made a huge difference in our grieving process.

I'm in the preparation room at the hospital, alone, as my partner stays in the waiting area. We were still in the midst of the COVID-19 situation, so partners weren't allowed to accompany us, even for this kind of situation.

The nurse approached and handed me two wrapped tablets. I've taken a lot of medication over the past three years, including many natural remedies. The sizes, colors, shapes, and packaging were all quite variable, but I had never seen a tablet so large and strangely wrapped in aluminum.

"Madam, here are your two medications to take before the procedure."

"Okay, what are they for?"

"One is acetaminophen for pain, and the other is to prevent side effects from the IV medications we'll be giving you. You can go to the bathroom to take them."

In the bathroom... I know it might seem ordinary to some people, but to me, this suppository was the pinnacle of my frustration. I've experienced a range of intense emotions over the past five days, the past three months, the past three years—could I catch a break?

I had a message in my SMS inbox.

— "Everything okay. Love?

— I just inserted a medication into an orifice that was supposed to be spared from any medical procedure in this process. I deserve to go eat ice cream at Walt Disney.

Minutes passed. What do you say to your girlfriend who, in such a crappy situation, gets hit with something as silly as inserting a suppository?

"I've bought the tickets. We're leaving tomorrow morning."

It might have seemed strange to want to grieve in a place crowded with children, where joy, wonder, and excitement were so palpable. But that's what I needed. I wanted to escape to another dimension. I wanted to experience intense emotions to try and revive in me, the light that had gone out a few days ago. I wanted to feel fear, scream, laugh, forget, and eat ice cream. With traces of opioids in my system, I attempted to pack a suitcase headed for "the most magical place on earth," under maternal supervision, as my mind remained in the icy room under the huge neon light facilitating the doctor's tunnel vision for the procedure.

Despite the endearing mascots, the dazzling parades, and the intoxicating ice creams, it was certain that an emotional storm was lurking very close to me. It was at the France pavilion, when a man dressed in period costume kindly explained to me that my favorite ride was unfortunately closed, that the lightning and thunder of my internal storm showed synchronicity. When Jean-François saw my face, he hugged me and tenderly said:

"Go ahead, let it out, that's why we're here."

And ironically, to the upbeat melody of Hakuna Matata in the background of Epcot's fireworks, I cried for my lost baby, cursing whoever may have forgotten to mention that Cinderella, Snow White, or Belle might not have had it easy before their happily ever after.

Several weeks passed. We tried our best to function at work and during our respective social events with our hearts still a little raw. It was a strange sensation to grieve for a soul we had never met. A few days later, we learned that our baby was not carrying a genetic anomaly such as Down syndrome. We were relieved but still had so many unanswered questions. Another inexplicable situation.

I sat on the floor in the hallway of our second floor in front of our four empty bedrooms. I still had some tears to shed. A mixture of sadness and gratitude filled me. The past three months had shown me the joy of mothering, and the desire to continue was still present and resonating in every cell of my body. Thousands of kilometers away from our home, an unjustified war was raging that would affect thousands of families. Jean-François came to join me:

"What would you say if we welcomed a Ukrainian family?"

I needed a project to take my mind off things. We were still grieving, but personally, I needed to occupy my brain because we were still facing a waiting period for the next steps in the process. Doctor's appointments, new tests to undergo, which would take several months before we got the results, and maybe moving on to a third transfer. Simply helping a family in need made me feel like I was embodying my desire to nurture. A completely selfish choice. Within a few weeks, through social media, we found a family of four Ukrainians who were in the process of moving to Quebec. We managed to get some information from a distant family friend about the who, when, how, and why, but even that sparse information was enough for us to jump into this adventure. It was a completely impulsive decision, guided by an emotionally unstable state, of which I was fully aware. Many found us intense, naive, and crazy to embark on such a significant project. For some, it was utterly absurd to voluntarily share our multigenerational home with strangers from a completely different culture. They accused us of mental alienation and labeled it "how to destroy your relationship 101." Others said it was an excellent way to "stop thinking about it," as we were reminded when we bought our house, when we adopted our dog... but in vain.

In spring 2022, all our energies were focused on integrating our Ukrainian family into our country. There were multiple forms to fill out, applications for various programs, fun French learning sessions, and simply helping them understand how our province works (which, looking back, was far from simple) ... In short, we had very little mental space left to think about our fertility process. And it did wonders for us. I had even managed to forget about the phone call with my doctor to announce that the results of my endometrial biopsy, hysteroscopy, and our genetic karyotype were all normal. Once our new summer routine with eight family members was well established, we saw the opportunity to proceed with the third embryo transfer. Over the next ten days after the procedure, I plunged into a state of "bodily hypervigilance." I analyzed every physical sensation because, unlike all the other times, I knew now, how to recognize the signs of pregnancy. I hated seeing myself like that. I was trapped in my thoughts, and no amount of lengthy government paperwork could set me free. On the morning of the blood test, I still had that damn bad feeling, and despite all the hope I placed on the occasional cramps and nausea felt here and there post-transfer, the result turned out negative. Tears, screams, disappointment, rage, incomprehension, and so on! Now, only one embryo remained.

November 2022, the moment of our last and final transfer. I had several months to prepare. For this last transfer, I couldn't afford any mistakes. I wanted to take action on my fertility. I wanted to be ready, to be at the peak of my physical and mental health. I wanted to prioritize myself and, above all, prioritize my greatest wish. For a few months, I worked hard on myself; I joined women's circles that helped me grow; I sought counsel. I talked. I wrote. I healed. I grew. I visualized. I was greatly apprehensive about the waiting period, hoping not to relive the same distress as during the third transfer. Forty-eight hours after the procedure, we left for Florida to join Jean-François's family. I would nurture this last embryo in the sun, and I hoped this escapade would divert my brain, which was slowly starting to analyze every cramp again. Despite my meditations, acupressure sessions, and Qi gong exercises to calm my anxiety and promote implantation, I experienced emotional bipolarity in the absence of symptoms one morning and the onset of a massive nausea in the evening. I tried to focus on the fact that I was surrounded by my loving in-laws, who treated me like a queen and never ceased to remind me of their love during one of my famous crying episodes. We returned the day before the pregnancy test appointment. I didn't want to wait because if the result turned out negative, I wanted as much time as possible to digest this blow. I took the urine test and, with trembling hands, immediately flipped the stick to hide the result. Jean-François read the test and confirmed it was negative. A wave of déjà vu washed over me. I was paralyzed by the despair that engulfed me. Once my brain had assessed the gravity of the situation, I collapsed to the floor, hitting it repeatedly with all my might while letting out screams of animosity that even surprised me. After exhausting my vocal cords and bruising my palm, I fell into a lethargic state. The invisible pain inside me was so unbearable that I had only one desire, to disappear. That's what I kept repeating to Jean-François, who, panicked to see me react like this, carried me to our bed, fearing I might start hitting the cold ceramic floor with all my strength again. He nestled against my back, and I could feel the tremor of his chest stifling deep sobs. I was aware of the seriousness of my words; I understood they could be interpreted as a desire to harm myself, in more ways than the bruises from hitting the bathroom floor. I was just exhausted from reliving the same disastrous scenario; I didn't think I had the strength to go through all the damn stages of grieving for the bundle of cells that had filled us with hope once again. I just fantasized about stopping feeling anything. The next day, Jean-François dragged me into the forest to clear our muddled minds. We talked, we cried, we screamed, and we dared to question what was next. Did we want a next step? Had we reached our limit? For me, that infamous limit was crossed the day I decided to embark on this winding journey of assisted reproduction. Instead, I wanted to listen to my inner voice that wanted to move forward, buoyed by whatever ounce of strength I had left.

With a lot of hindsight, today I am able to feel gratitude for our fertility journey. If I had the choice, I would certainly have chosen an easier, quicker path with the certainty of a final destination. However, I would not have taken the time to stop and realize the inner strength that resides within me, guiding me towards realizing my dream of becoming a mother one day. These past four years have made me realize how powerful, resilient, tolerant, and patient a woman can be. On the eve of my third in vitro fertilization (yes, third), I thank whatever spiritual entity allows me to continue to rely on the support, love, and comfort of my partner. While this adventure could have cost us our relationship several times, we have decided, nonetheless, to make it our strength. Becoming a mother comes with its own set of challenges, and for me, my journey to motherhood extends far beyond the moment when I will hold our miracle in my arms. I must recognize it, accept it, breathe, and continue to move forward.

CHAPTER 7

THE PATH TO LIFE DONORS

By Nadine Mailloux

Her little footsteps echoed down the corridor, and a cherubic face with eyes like a beautiful blue sky met mine, halfway open:

— "Mommy! My Peppa Pig plush fell under my bed, and I can't reach it!

— Shh, Mia, you're too loud, lower your voice.

— But, Mommy, I want my plush and some cereal."

It's 6:45 in the morning, and her father and I are on holiday. I feel a bit irritated to be woken up by this little voice, far too enthusiastic for this early hour, but... there are mornings when I remember that this blonde little girl, who will soon be 4 years old, is a gift we almost didn't receive.

2014

I'm in the midst of separating from my partner, all the while taking full-time care of our two children. As an only child, raised by separated parents from a tender age and with a father who was rarely present, my deepest desire was to create a harmonious and loving family unit. In my mind, I kept asking myself, "Why? Why didn't I see the inevitable cracks sooner?"

When you have a clear dream of what you want your family life to be like and that dream is shattered, your heart feels like it's dying inside. While I was suffering from this failure, I had to move on, for the sake of my little ones, who were then barely

3 and 5 years old. I left the relationship with a deep fear of the unknown, of the repercussions that loom on the horizon, haunted by the specter of retaliation that could wreak havoc on us all. In the depths of my mind, a thought echoed relentlessly: "How can I ever hope to piece together the fragments of our shattered family? What kind of mother does that make me?"

I struggled to recover from this ordeal, perhaps one of the most challenging experiences I had ever confronted. I had to mourn my cherished family ideal, a painful reminder of unfulfilled promises. Fueled by bitterness and sorrow, I embarked on a journey towards happiness, though at the time, it felt impossible to achieve. Like many others, I was on the verge of depression. Alcohol and tears were part of my life when the children went away every other weekend.

Fortunately, adversity often brings self-discovery and renewal. In fact, my dearest friend of twenty years went through an equally painful separation just three months after mine. It was through our tumultuous love stories that we found each other in a way we never expected. With the gentle encouragement of a friend and hesitant steps into the realm of dating, our paths began to converge. That's when our friendship blossomed into something altogether unexpected. A love that had always been there, dormant beneath the surface, finally revealed itself in all its raw authenticity.

2015

It didn't take me long to realize that I wanted this remarkable and caring man, who showered such love and attention on my two young children, to also become the father of our future child. Even before our romantic relationship began, I made him a heartfelt promise: "If you're open to it, I'd love nothing more than to build a family together, filled with plenty of children."

From a young age, I held a clear vision in my heart—the dream of nurturing a large and loving family. However, a significant obstacle shadowed over this dream: his severe fertility issue. This reality became apparent during his previous relationship, where he attempted to conceive for the first time. When he first shared the diagnosis—OATS, or oligo-astheno-teratozoospermia—with me, I needed him to repeat it, then immediately turned to the internet for answers. In simple terms, this condition meant that his sperm count was low, their motility poor, and their shape abnormal. According to the doctor, his chance of conceiving naturally was a mere 0.00001%, an almost insurmountable hurdle. Despite these daunting odds, my determination remained unchallenged. I held onto my dream of expanding our family, of rebuilding what had been lost, alongside a partner who shared my deepest values. Within just a month of being together, I was resolute in my desire to conceive a child with my best friend of twenty years. The thought of him never experiencing fatherhood was inconceivable to me. Meanwhile, we took practical steps to prepare for the future. We sold my old house and renovated our basement, ensuring that my two precious children, aged 4 and 6, felt safe and comfortable in their new surroundings. Their wellbeing was crucial, especially considering the turmoil they had experienced in the past year. What made our relocation particularly special was my mother's suggestion to bury a statue of St. Joseph upside down in the flower bed of my old home. An old tale meant to expedite the sale and alleviate my financial burdens. With her guidance, we followed this tradition, and to our amazement, an offer to purchase the house came just days later. I closed the sale between Christmas and New Year's Day, marking the start of a fresh chapter for me and my beloved children.

THE BEGINNING OF THE PROCESS

"Good morning, Mrs. Mailloux, you and your partner will meet with Dr. Speedy Gonzales at the hospital in one month." (This nickname was bestowed upon him following this first meeting, for our fertility specialist is a gentleman who comes in like a whirlwind, explains everything at lightning speed, and then leaves just as quickly). I hung up the phone, my heart racing with excitement, and immediately texted my partner to share the good news: our first appointment is finally scheduled. Little do I know at that moment; it marks only the beginning of a journey that will span several years. Along the way, we will encounter a roller coaster of emotions—from anticipation and hope to moments of despair and doubt. Our path will be marked by shattered illusions, financial sacrifices, and countless moments of waiting that seem to stretch on endlessly. But through it all, we will also find moments of unexpected joy, unwavering support, and ultimately, acceptance.

We've been sitting in the office for 15 minutes now, and we waited at least 30 minutes in the waiting room. I'm already stressed about being late for work because I'm not a regular employee and I'm already on borrowed time.

— "Seriously, honey, do you think it's going to take much longer? I haven't told my colleagues why I'll be late this morning.

— I have no idea. I also have important appointments waiting for me."

It's at this moment that Dr. Speedy Gonzales enters the office in a whirlwind. He greets us with a smile, rummages through his files, looks at us, and says:

"Well, madam, you've already had two children without difficulty, you're still young (33 years old at this time), so everything should go well. You've had blood tests to check your AMH, prolactin, and FSH. Your thyroid is a bit high, so I'm going to prescribe medication for that, and we'll need to redo blood tests to check your prolactin. Your last gynecological exam is not up to date. I can do it for you now if you want."

My partner and I look a bit lost in the face of so much information in such a short time. The doctor continues:

"And you, sir, I see that you have severe OATS, so the chances of success with insemination are very slim, if not impossible. Have you considered the option of donors? I've seen many couples over the years, and their children all look like them!"

My partner responds that he hadn't considered this option and that we want to try IVF. The doctor adds:

"As you wish, but I'm telling you, no one can guess they don't carry the same genes."

Oops! The doctor probably didn't mean any harm and is just trying to find the option with the highest chances of success for everyone, but my sweetheart doesn't really agree with his words. We end the meeting with our tests to undergo and our file sent to a private clinic for in vitro fertilization. As we leave the clinic, I sense my partner feeling tense and irritated (which is not like him at all).

"Did you hear how casually he threw out the option of donors? As if it were nothing! He's never been through any of this himself, so how can he say it's normal to consider a donor?" From that moment on, this option was no longer part of our discussions.

Embarking on fertility procedures feels like venturing into uncharted territory. You don't know the terms, the next steps, or the timelines involved. As someone naturally inclined towards impatience, I had to learn the art of breathing through it all. In this journey, waiting becomes a constant companion. Waiting for appointment dates, enduring long waits at appointments (often running an hour late), awaiting the arrival of day one, anxiously anticipating test results, and holding our breath to see if we've finally achieved conception... But the waiting doesn't end there. There are lost results, tests needing retakes, and moments when I hang up the phone, tears streaming down my cheeks, or muttering curses under my breath, exhausted by the never-ending stream of obstacles, delays, and tests. Why all these tests?" I often wonder, frustrated by the barrage of medical scrutiny. "I'm fertile, aren't I?" And yet, month after month, we find ourselves back at square one, our lives suspended in a perpetual cycle of uncertainty. Meanwhile, our relatives, though well-intentioned, often fumble in the dark, struggling to comprehend the depths of our struggle. Being told not to stress or not to think about it feels like a slap in the face. How can I not think about it when every day is filled with reminders—three pills to take, night sweats from side effects, work hours rearranged for ultrasound appointments, and so on? My partner sometimes felt useless and uncomfortable seeing me go through all this when he was "the problem." At each stage, he offers me an out, reassuring me that I'm free to stop anytime. In fact, many people told me, "You must really love him to put yourself through all this," or "Why are you doing all this when you already have two children?"

The truth is, I entered this journey with a clear vision: to become a parent alongside him and to provide my two older children with the example of a united family. The decision was mine alone, and despite the well-meaning comments from others questioning my choices, I remained anchored in my position. This journey isn't just about us; it's about the countless individuals who, month after month, continue to chase their own miracles. Their lives, their choices — they are not up for debate or commentary from those who cannot fathom the depths of their struggle. In the end, it's about finding strength in the face of adversity and holding onto hope, even when the path ahead seems clouded in darkness.

Starting a fertility journey is like stepping into a storm of emotions: you know when it starts, but you have no idea when it will be over. Sometimes the clouds fade to let a few rays of sunshine through, and in an instant, the dark clouds come back rushing in. There's also the tornado that can wreak havoc in no time. It's like jumping feet first into the void, hoping to land with a baby in your arms. My sweetheart went through many storms before accepting his fertility issue. He took the initiative to be accompanied by a sex therapist to better navigate the ordeal we were facing. I believe men are less supported in this matter than women, and the subject is still very taboo.

2016

As our paperwork finally came together, I eagerly counted down the days to our first appointment like a child awaiting a special occasion. The private clinic was a two-hour journey from our home. However, with only a short-term contract as a specialized educator and minimal vacation time, this marked the beginning of "vacations on my own dime"—a source of added stress due to the financial strain. Alongside the logistical challenges, there was the constant juggle of arranging childcare for my two older children, who resided with us almost full-time. Co-parenting complexities added another layer of tension, as my ex-partner and I struggled to find common ground on various matters concerning them. Despite two years without requesting shared custody, their father suddenly expressed readiness, conflicting with our desired custody arrangement based on our beliefs and values.

In the midst of our IVF journey, we encountered significant personal setbacks. Tragically, my partner's mother, battling a lung infection for years, passed away during our treatments. This loss deeply affected us, causing a pause in our momentum as my partner took time off work to grieve. Despite the emotional toll, we remained steadfast in our commitment to each other, emerging from the ordeal stronger and more united as a couple.

With a whirlwind of emotions swirling within us, we embarked on a marathon journey that would span years. Though we held onto hope, there lingered a cloud of apprehension about what lay ahead. As we made the journey to the clinic, I clasped my partner's hand, offering reassurance, "We'll have our little miracle, my love." His response, a heartfelt affirmation, reflected his own fervent desire for our shared dream.

Upon our arrival at the clinic, I found the wait terribly long and the waiting room depressing. The initial encounter with the doctor only added to the solemnity, as he presented our options with clinical detachment. It was evident that we were just another couple navigating the labyrinth of fertility challenges. He had seen couples like us countless times before:

— "Given the high quality of your eggs, we will only need a few sperm that the embryologist will select based on their quality. So, your best option is IVF ICSI.

— Can you remind me, what is ICSI?"

He explained to us that with this procedure, a sperm would be injected into each mature follicle they found during the egg retrieval. Additionally, I would need to take medication to stimulate the production of as many follicles as possible, along with another medication to trigger ovulation. We left the appointment that day filled with hope, armed with a statistic—approximately a 25% chance of success.

Since all the terms used during the appointment seemed complex to me, I began researching them on the internet. That's when I also discovered a community on Facebook for people facing fertility issues. I was able to ask all my questions and gain a deeper understanding thanks to these individuals. Yet, it was also there that I sometimes felt like an impostor because I already had children. This feeling followed me everywhere, whether in the hospital waiting room or when discussing the ongoing procedures with close friends and family. People would say, "You must really love him to endure all this! Besides, you already have two kids." What these individuals didn't understand was that I wanted this baby just as much as my partner did, and I was willing to do whatever it took to make it happen. Of course, it was about deep love, respect, and the desire to give this gift to such a wonderful man, but it was also about becoming a mother with him and imparting our shared values to a little one.

THE INJECTIONS FOR THE FIRST IVF

After carefully listening to the nurse's instructions on how to use the injections, my partner and I left feeling stressed and excited at the same time.

— "Honey? Honey?"

My partner calls out to me from our bedroom because he managed to prepare the mixture for our first injection, the first of many.

— "Just a moment, I'm turning on the TV for the kids"

Finding a moment of 'peace' for ourselves before the kids, aged 6 and 8, headed off to school was quite challenging. We were keeping all of this a secret from them because they were too young to understand. So, it added an extra layer of stress, and my partner was afraid of hurting me or not injecting enough medication. I remember once, he had prepared everything in our room and had called me over. I quickly settled the kids and hurried to join him. He barely had time to touch my stomach to administer the injection when the youngest started crying. I had to step out to calm things down while my partner held the syringe ready to inject me. I still remember his cold, trembling fingers as he held onto my belly to administer the injection. At the same time, it was almost the only power he had in all of this. He wasn't the one burdened with mental load, dealing with appointments for ultrasounds that made me wait an hour while I had to go to work and the side effects of the medication (though, yes, he endured my sometimes-difficult mood). I do believe he must have felt even worse since he was the one with fertility issues, and I was the one undergoing the treatments.

To keep our relationship on track, we talked a lot about our emotions throughout all of this. We tried to take it one day at a time, but I was always making plans or thinking about the next step. "Well, if I calculate and have my egg retrieval on such a date, I'll be able to take such a day off. If I get pregnant after, I'll be off work and have a decent amount of parental leave, but if it's in three months, it will be more difficult..." With time, I don't remember all the results from my multiple ultrasound appointments, but I remember the waiting and the stress it caused. When you embark on this process, you're filled with hope, your heart swollen with courage, and that's what keeps you going. However, the outcome remains unknown until you reach the ultimate goal of this journey. From our perspective, all the doctors and nurses we met were confident in our chances of success. I was still young at 33, had no fertility issues, and they needed the best sperm to inject into my eggs. So, on the big day, we set off for the clinic two hours away telling ourselves that everything would be fine, trying to ignore the feeling of the unknown that lingered.

THE RETRIEVAL

Due to severe insomnia that had been persisting for months, I decided to take the sleeping medication I had been prescribed. I felt fragile and was still experiencing a lot of stress related to my ex-partner and our children. I was desperately trying to find a way to make their lives easier and softer, but I had no control over their father's violent behaviors and reactions. I was constantly in a state of hypervigilance and worry. Fortunately, I was seeing professionals to help me move forward in all of this. Additionally, my partner and my family were also there for me.

So, on the morning of the egg retrieval, I woke up very early. "Well, finally the big day, what will happen? Will it hurt? What if I don't have enough follicles..." My partner held me close in bed before we started this day, and I saw my own mixed emotions, mirrored in him, between worry and excitement. Since we had to get there quite early, we cut short our embrace. Usually of calm demeanor, my partner, that morning, seemed stressed and with a concerned tone, said:

— "I hope I abstained long enough! What if they don't find any? I hope it goes well during the retrieval!" After all, he was the one who had to retreat to a private room for the delicate task of producing semen to ensure a successful procedure. The pressure he felt was palpable, and I couldn't help but sympathize with the weight of responsibility resting on his shoulders. That morning, I was grateful not to be in his position.

Once settled, a doctor I didn't know entered accompanied by his intern, a medical apprentice of whom I was unaware. I gave them the go ahead, and with my whole small womanly body (I'm 5 feet 1 inch tall and weighed 110 pounds at the time), I let the four needles enter my cervix to numb it and make it less painful. I had given birth twice, but I had never prepared myself for this sharp and surprising pain. That was just the beginning because the retrieval itself tore me away from the unicorn world I had been living in since the beginning of these procedures. My partner held my hand, attempting to impart some of his strength, yet he couldn't take my place in that chair. The intern gave up and let the doctor finish the job because I couldn't bear being poked around in my lower abdomen while suffering excruciating pain. As far as I remember, our first harvest was the best of all: fourteen follicles!

— "Phew! Darling! I think we didn't go through all of this for nothing.

— I truly hope so. Know that If I could I would have taken your pain as my own.

— Don't worry, I'll be ok. The important thing is to have a beautiful embryo to transfer."

Some time later, a nurse came to inform us that eleven follicles had been micro-injected, and we would know in the coming days if life was developing. The longest and most stressful days: those when you wait for the famous call from the embryologist to tell you how things are going. Clearly, that's not when my sleep improved.

DAY 1

7:00 AM, the phone rings. I dart towards it as if my life depends on it, while my mind conjures up ten scenarios simultaneously.

"Yes, hello."

"Good morning, Mrs. Mailloux, it's the embryologist."

At that moment, I try to discern from the tone of his voice whether he has good or bad news to deliver.

"On your eleven micro-injected eggs, only two high-quality embryos are currently developing."

"Only two? How is that possible?"

"Several factors may come into play, including the issue with your partner."

"Are our chances still good?"

"We will let the two embryos rest until tomorrow, and we will give you an update on day 3 to see if a transfer is possible."

I hang up, and my throat tightens... I can only think of the two embryos. It's so little. My partner also thought it was few, but with his natural optimism, he had helped me keep hope alive:

"If they kept them, it means they have a chance, so I think we should focus on that."

DAY 3

The news seems somewhat good as we are asked to come in on this fateful day 3 for the transfer of the 2 embryos that apparently have a chance of implantation.

"Yes, hello."

"Mrs. Mailloux, it's the clinic. We have decided to transfer both embryos at the same time to increase your chances of pregnancy."

"Okay, so we're not waiting any longer to see their development?"

"Based on their number of cells, we believe this is the best option."

I didn't understand why they were transferring both embryos either. I was left with a bitter taste in my mouth because I always had this feeling that I wasn't being told the whole truth and that our chances weren't as high as they seemed.

"Honey! Come see, we see a line, is it possible so soon?"

"What! I see it too," he replied, his eyes sparkling.

Ultimately, this happiness only lasted for a day. After that, we did our research and learned that the medication that triggers ovulation can also leave visible traces on pregnancy tests. So, after the infamous negative blood test, we were back to square one.

FIV #2

Two months later, we had some savings set aside, and I had a very concrete goal: to have a baby with my partner. So, back to medications, same protocol, ultrasounds, and all that jazz. Amidst work, children, and the stresses of daily life, we were back at it. Confident, still full of hope and excitement, my partner asked me:

— "Are you sure you want to start again now?

— Yes, absolutely sure. Since we're in this, let's go for it and we'll get our gift of life".

Unfortunately, even with eleven mature follicles retrieved, one embryo transferred, and none frozen, that gift didn't arrive then.

— "Honey, I'm taking you on a trip!"

I'm at work, calling my partner. I've decided we're going down south... in the middle of summer!

— "How? What?"

I can sense doubt in his voice. He's definitely not the spontaneous type, so I try to convince him over the phone that this is the best decision ever.

— "Trust me, it'll work out. I want to go and enjoy the sun with you, I've never been there, and we need a little break.

— But with what money? We can't really afford it right now.

— Let's talk about it tonight, don't worry about the details, I've got it all figured out".

The following week, we had booked a one-week trip to Mexico. I was over the moon, finally escaping home to a warm destination. Yet, organizing the trip was quite a task, considering we had two kids; leaving them for a week wasn't that simple. Especially since, at that time, they were almost always with us. After our initial FIV failure, we needed this time to reconnect. Fortunately, my savings allowed us to venture far. However, the stress of our journey tagged along. The Zika virus loomed in Mexico, and fertility clinics strongly advised against travel to prevent infection, citing potential harm to a future baby and the apparent danger. Upon our return, we even lied to the nurses about our recent travels.

— "Have you traveled in the past few months? As you may know, the Zika virus is circulating in several countries and can lead to congenital malformations..."

I'm looking at my partner, silently begging him to keep quiet. It's really not his style to lie. Fortunately, he replied:

— "No, not at all."

So, we decided to go anyway, but with a cloud hanging over our heads, the intense worry of being bitten by a ravaging mosquito. I still remember one particular time when it was extremely hot with humidity in the air. We were returning from a lavish evening with ample alcoholic beverages and were in a small transport cart at the resort. I needed to use the restroom, so we got off the vehicle in a darker spot with a tiny light. That attracted hundreds of thirsty mosquitoes.

— "Hurry up! There are lots of mosquitoes and we mustn't get bitten," my partner told me.

Panic sets in, and even with a bottle of mosquito repellent applied to my body, the tiny Zika-infected insects were after me.

I can't remember if I took the time to urinate in the end or if I just grabbed my partner's hand and said:

— "Quick, we have to leave!"

We constantly feared the worst, worrying our baby project would come to a stop. I think my partner was more cautious than me in such situations. Yet, given the significant investment we made, we desperately needed some sense of relief.

FIV #3

After the disappointment and discouragement of our last two attempts, we had to decide on the next steps. Our lives were filled with hardships at that moment. On one hand, my partner's mother passed away from a lung disease she had been battling for years. On the other, I had to cope with the change from almost full custody to shared custody with the father of my children, alternating weeks. When you're going through fertility treatments, life doesn't stop. Everything else happening around you is adding an extra layer of stress.

— "I think it would be a viable alternative to retrieve sperm directly from the testicles. It will most likely allow for better quality," the doctor at the clinic mentioned during a visit before our next IVF attempt. "With this technique, the odds will be on your side, but the efficacy can only be confirmed once we retrieve them from the source"

This is when my partner came up with a new word: *testiballs.*

He still bears the mark from this procedure, and so do I, as it was the worst of the three FIV attempts.

ULTIMATE RETRIEVAL

It's morning; I'm stressed; my body is stiff; I'm uncertain of our choice. My partner is going to provide a sample of semen, just before the retrieval. He accompanies me, as he always does, into the cold room, and I put my feet in the stirrups. I'm there with my intimacy wide open. I wait, until I feel the needle stick four times in my cervix. They talk to me, but I don't hear anymore; I just want a good harvest, at last. Unfortunately, it was the worst of all.

— "How many eggs do we have?" I ask impatiently to the nurse who came to check on me.

— "Nine mature ones," she replies.

— "Just that? It's so few...

— You only need one embryo to succeed; I've seen much smaller harvests result in a baby," she says to encourage me. "Now, I have to leave and go with your partner for his procedure."

It's the weekend, the doctor had to bring her child because she cut her vacation short to perform our procedures. She leaves him with me after my retrieval, heading to an operating room where

I can't be. Finally, they come to see me after almost an hour of waiting alone with this child and my feeling of emptiness.

— "And?

— It's not the result we hoped for: only a few low-quality sperm.

— What?"

My partner just suffered like never before, just for this? How is this possible? What an injustice! I'm angry at life for doing this to us after so much time, energy, and money invested. In the end, no viable embryo developed, and we're back to square one. My partner was discouraged, and I was already in problem-solving mode.

THE PATH TO LIFE DONORS

— "What if we looked at sperm donor websites, to better understand how it works? As an informational step... It is not binding us to anything..."

I had secretly been contemplating this option for quite some time. I couldn't fathom that everything was coming to an end, not after the journey we'd been through. "I'm not sure if I'm ready for this option," was his initial response, but I sensed some openness. So, I gave him the time and space he needed to think about it. Meanwhile, he continued to share his thoughts with a sex therapist. I still recall the butterflies I felt in my stomach the day he announced that he had embraced this option as well.

In the meantime, we had to make sure that all my tests were up to date, which also took a few months. We were required to meet with a psychologist who thought it wasn't a good idea to embark on this adventure. Nevertheless, we took a leap of faith.

— "The psychologist thinks we have too much on our plates, but I am confident that we will manage. What do you think?

— I think we should continue. We'll see how we feel every step of the way, like we've done before. Even though it's a lot of stress, it's about life. It's so positive and happy that it will only soothe the pain of losing my mother.

The search for someone who could help us become parents felt very different at first. We screened all kinds of faces, qualities, genetic issues, and health backgrounds. It's very easy to get lost in it, and my husband had very strict criteria. The most important thing: he had to inspire confidence and be an open donor, meaning he accepted that our child, upon turning 18, could contact him if they wanted to. After some time, we found him. He was the "guy" we needed. We would still incur fees, but we were ready to take that risk. We were all in, like when playing poker.

— "Look honey, he has that smart look, just like you, what do you think?

— Yeah, it's true, he's got the same vibe as me. Plus, he's tall and has blue eyes.

— So, should we go for it?

— There's no guarantee, but let's order and see.

— How about taking three samples, it's cheaper for delivery."

I felt both excited and stressed. Would we find the winning recipe this time around? I don't remember much about the first two inseminations, but I remember very well the disappointment and sadness we felt. Discouragement was starting to weigh heavily on our shoulders. It had been nearly three years since we had been waiting for our little miracle to grow inside my belly. My mother thought I was overdoing it:

— "Maybe you should stop all this. You already have enough with two to take care of. It can't be good either to take all these hormones in the long run. I know you want your husband to become a father, but you shouldn't wear yourself out.

— No, Mom, I can't stop now. It's going to happen, you'll see."

We're in the hospital elevator. We just experienced the most unusual insemination.

— "I can't believe we just went through that. This has got to be the bottom of the barrel. I bet you this time it's going to work!"

Looking back on this last insemination, it feels like a bad comedy movie. While the nurse held our last sample, she accidentally spilled some of it into the paper where the syringe was and had to pump it back in:

— "Oh no, some of the sample spilled out of the syringe!"

I looked at my partner, in complete disbelief.

— "It's okay, I managed to put it back in."

As if it wasn't stressful enough, the doctor had to inseminate me twice because there was still some left in the syringe.

— "Well, if it works, it's because that child really wanted to be here."

On that first day after my period was due, I took a pregnancy test, knowing deep inside me that the long awaited second line would finally appear! I was so excited and happy that I cried tears of joy. In fact, it's the only time throughout our journey that I managed to wait before testing. Our daughter was born perfectly healthy at thirty-eight weeks of pregnancy, and she's now four years old. She really wanted to be here. She fills our family with her presence.

2023, ONE LAST ONE, HONEY?

Finally, I have the nurse's approval to start the progesterone after my morning ultrasound. It's been three months already that we've been waiting for the transfer of our one and only frozen embryo on day 5. I'm in a strange state: "Should I be happy, full of hope, or simply in a state of letting go and detachment? I feel mixed between all these ways of approaching what will happen in the coming days. I had told my partner that using a donor for IVF was our last attempt and that if it didn't work, we would 'close the shop' and move on. I still hear myself saying to the nurse:

'What! Only nine eggs retrieved? Only five mature?' But I wasn't on my first attempt, and the naivety was gone. I knew very well that out of five, few or none continue their development to reach day 5. Although our relationship is strong, my partner cannot experience everything happening in my body, and sometimes I am in a terrible mood. I'm tired, and even sick of all these appointments, this waiting, these hopes, and disappointments, but at the same time, reaching the end without having that little being growing inside me frustrates me enormously. She had been kind and had tried to encourage me by saying that it was not the quantity but the quality that mattered. The days after the retrieval are endless. You're there, staring at your phone every two minutes, waiting for the long-awaited call from the embryologist. You go through fifty thousand scenarios, and in the end, none of them come true. Finally, after five days, two embryos were in the race, one of which, apparently, was of good quality, a 4bb grade. It was the one they transferred to me first. Bang! First failure, after my breasts had swollen for a few days for nothing. In the infertility jargon, they call it a biochemical miscarriage. Many women experience it, without necessarily knowing they do. My second one in six months. I was starting to think that my eggs were old and dried up.

I don't know if I'll have the strength to continue if this last little spark of life doesn't hold on. At my age (thirty-nine years old), I should focus again on myself and my life as a woman and a wife, not only as a mom, especially since I already have three who still demand a lot from me. Why insist on having another one at all costs? What motivates all these women to push their bodies and minds to the limit to become mothers? In the end, is it just a primal instinct? Or is it a need so strong and powerful that when it's not fulfilled, it's a lack that is felt for the rest of one's life? And what about "cases" like mine? I'm sure many women struggling with infertility will resent me for not being satisfied after three attempts when they have been waiting for motherhood for so long.

That infamous day 1 has arrived, the one we dread or hope for. In my case, I awaited it with a mixture of eagerness and impatience.

— "Hi, this is Julie, the nurse from the clinic. We can't find the results of your cytology. It says here that it has expired."

A slight wave of panic begins to sweep over me. I'm two weeks away from the FET that I've been waiting for three long months. It's impossible for me to wait another month to redo an exam they forgot to have me retake.

— "I don't understand. I remember having one before my IVF in October.

— I can't find it in your file. We'll need to double-check because it needs to be up to date.

— Okay, but what do I do? I only have two weeks to sort this out, and you know, it's not just my exams that are expired. My fertility isn't far from expiring either."

I tried a joke to lighten the mood, but it seems she didn't find me funny because she continues:

— "You need this exam, maybe ask the nurses to perform it externally for you.

I find myself once again chasing exams and appointments, wondering why they couldn't have informed me three months ago. It's frustrating, but I immediately call the nurse, who assures me it's fine to come in the next morning. After all that stress, I'm told my results are up to date, but I still need to provide a urine sample for another matter that should have been handled. Phew... So here I am on day 13 for my ultrasound. How many ultrasounds has there been since the beginning? Twenty? Thirty? Well, it's hard to keep count, but there have been quite a few. I'm given the green light to start another medication, vaginal progesterone three times a day, which supposedly increases my chances of success, though it serves as a reminder that none of this is very natural. I return to work, attending to the lively needs of the children, with my other three waiting for me at home in the evening. There's no time to overthink. At least, that's what I tell myself. Sometimes, I let my mind wander, imagining having another baby to cuddle and care for, with our almost four-year-old daughter helping me. Then I snap back to reality, to the statistics, and to the last failed attempts. When I share my feelings with my husband, he remains his positive self, encouraging me to do the same. Finally, on day 13, I have an ultrasound, and everything looks good. I text my husband, who has been eagerly awaiting the transfer date to plan his work leave. As a social worker, rearranging appointments is complicated, and there's no one to replace him. We decided to take some time for ourselves by spending a night in Quebec City. Almost eight years of love for both of us. Almost thirty years since we've known each other. In the end, we obtained a total of two embryos, only two. One of them was transferred to me on day 5, supposedly of good quality, but it didn't result in anything. The other was implanted three months later, without high expectations, and unfortunately, it didn't attach either.

AWARENESS IS KEY

I have always believed that we should start with the young to sensitize them about a subject or a process. Perhaps it's due to my profession and that of my partner that we immediately decided to share our choice to have a child with the help of a donor with the whole family. My eldest was just twelve years old when I explained to her how her little sister came into our lives. We were enjoying a mother-daughter spa activity, finally allowing for some one-on-one time with her, away for any kind of distractions.

I cherish these moments with my now almost fourteen-year-old daughter because it feels like we can finally have open conversations without any barriers. So, one evening, as we settled in comfortably together, she said:

— "Mom, I was doing some research on my phone and I saw on Google that it said donor bank."

I hadn't expected my daughter to come across that google search, and I wanted to wait until I was with my partner to explain it all to her. It was at that moment that I saw her intelligent eyes fixed on me, waiting for a clear and precise answer.

— "Do you know that Yan and I are trying to have another child?

— Yes, I know.

— We're searching for a man who can help us succeed, like we did for your sister.

— Are you saying that my sister isn't Yan's daughter?

— If you only knew, my love... where do I begin?"

And that's when I told her, in a condensed version, everything we had gone through before her sister came into our lives. In our family values, it was essential that our daughter knew where she came from and how she came to be with us. There would be no secrets, and we wanted to keep an open discussion about her genetic background. Both of my eldest children had to know the truth about their little sister's story so that everything would be transparent and sincere. Thus, as she grows older, she'll understand just how much she was cherished, anticipated, and yearned for.

CHAPTER 8

BEYOND INFERTILITY

By Genevieve Fillion

I"m pleased to meet you; my name is Geneviève. It's March 2023. I'm 32 years old and I'm caught in the whirlwind of infertility, like many other women across the world. I hope that as you read these lines, you'll find solace in knowing you're not alone. These words have been saved on the Notes app of my phone over countless moments, penned with the depth of my soul. With unfiltered honesty, I share my journey with you, drawing from the raw emotions that reside within me. Let me begin by recounting the foundation of our love story. It all started on Tinder, where I stumbled upon a profile of a brown-haired man with captivating blue eyes, and fate led us to match. From July to September of 2019, we conversed virtually, slowly building a connection that intrigued me enough to suggest we meet in person. We met after my shift, at a local bar. As I waited outside, he arrived, his smile lighting up the night. He was so handsome, I had butterflies in my stomach. Seated together, within mere seconds, I sensed deep within me that he was destined to be the father of my children.

In the following months, we cautiously navigated our budding relationship, with me maintaining guarded walls around my heart. Then, in March 2020, serendipity led us both to Asia, where our paths converged once more. What began as a solo journey for each of us transformed into a shared adventure filled with love. However, our bliss was cut short by the pandemic, compelling us to return home urgently. We decided to spend our mandatory isolation in my apartment. Despite contracting COVID-19, this is where our bond deepened. Only two months had passed, but our love for one another was so strong that it felt as if we had lived a lifetime together. As our love blossomed, discussions about starting a family naturally arose. Alexandre suffered from cancer in his early twenties, so we knew he was infertile. Despite his strong apprehensions, my love for him knew no bounds, and the prospect of conceiving through assisted means did not discourage me. Thus, I embraced the journey of infertility, unaware of what I was getting into or the challenges that lay ahead.

In September 2020, I had my first consultation at the fertility clinic, where the doctor elucidated the intricacies of insemination and the battery of tests awaiting me. Throughout the fall, I underwent a myriad of blood tests and ultrasounds, alongside diligently monitoring my ovulation with daily urine tests spanning ten days. Determining the optimal time for conception proved to be a far cry from the textbook theories, as it took three months to pinpoint the elusive moment—occurring on the 18th day of my cycle, defying conventional norms.

In January 2021, I embarked on my first natural cycle insemination, with a strong belief that success would come swiftly. Fueled by naivety and boundless hope, I returned home with unwavering optimism. That evening, our connection seemed to transcend, leading us to a profound intimacy unlike any before. An amusing anecdote arises from that moment—it unfolded in the basement of my in-laws' home. Typically lacking in privacy, this time, we were deep in our own bubble, oblivious to the surrounding noises. It wasn't until we found ourselves moving to the rhythm of my mother-in-law's disco music that we were sent back to reality. "1, 2, 3, go! Let's dance! The dance of love!" Alas, a few days later, my hopes were dashed as my period arrived unexpectedly, leaving me without even the chance to take a pregnancy test.

Then, I had another appointment with a new doctor at the same clinic. In February 2021, I had my second natural cycle insemination. Since it was during the pandemic, my partner had to stay in the car while the procedure took place in a small emotionless cardboard room. We were several women, separated by a curtain as if we were heading to the slaughterhouse. There was a lack of warmth. Three days later, panicked, in a pool of blood, I called the clinic. I wanted to know if it was normal. Unfortunately, the nurse told me that I had gotten my period more than a week early, and I thought I had had a miscarriage.

Afterwards, I had, once again, a new doctor. He decided to change the protocol. In March 2021, I had my third insemination, this time, based on a hormone cycle. It is when the chaos began.

The following month, I received a letter in the mail. My clinic was closing its doors, and our file was transferred elsewhere. I contacted the new clinic, and with that very first call, I could feel a much-improved customer-oriented approach. The summer of 2021 was difficult. We thought my partner's cancer had returned. He didn't want to undergo chemotherapy again. I thought I would support him emotionally through this stage. However, that wasn't the case. Slowly, the failures of the inseminations played in my head without me realizing it. At the end of the summer, we learned his bone marrow transplant was reacting to him having contracted COVID-19. However, after several months of heavy medication, he was starting to get better. To fill the void of unconditional love from a baby, we adopted a Sphynx cat. Instantly, I fell in love with him as if he were my human baby. I already had a street cat who was affectionate, but my Sphynx was THE cuddle monster I needed.

In September 2021, I was alone at home, on the phone with the doctor from the new clinic. It was at that moment that my heart stopped beating as if I had fallen from a twenty-story building. The doctor had analyzed my file transferred from the previous clinic. He bluntly revealed that I could never conceive through insemination, given my low ovarian reserve. This diagnosis had never been formulated before. The doctors had told me that everything was fine. That day, I found out that I too, had infertility problems.

Next step: IVF. And thus began the long wait! The infamous IVF waiting list... it's torture! Every month, periods come and go, and another cycle is lost.

In the meantime, bad news arrived. My father-in-law had terminal cancer. I wished so much to get the call confirming our turn had arrived and finally be able to announce to him that he might be a grandfather. It was his greatest wish. By Christmas 2021, I still hadn't heard from the clinic. The holidays passed alongside my in-laws, surrounded with unconditional love and building fond memories.

In March 2022, at last, that long-awaited call arrived. I started the injections with a lot of stress. Luckily, my partner wanted to administer them for me. I set an alarm on my phone for eight o'clock with baby emojis so I wouldn't miss the time. At the appointed hour, I prepared the medication. As a nurse by profession, handling medications in powder and water form was routine for me. But oh, the panic that ensued when I experienced a slight spillage of the mixture! When it's for yourself, even the smallest task can turn into a daunting challenge. Then came the moment I dreaded the most: the burning sensation of the hormone injection, unbearable each time. This medication had been part of all three of my IVF treatments, tarnishing my perception of injections. Thankfully, this painful moment always passed with the calm presence and encouragement of my loving partner.

Then came the first ultrasound, and for the second time, my heart seemed to stop beating. The doctor, without an ounce of empathy, delivered the crushing news that my cycle was to be canceled due to one follicle being "too large." It was a possibility I had never imagined, and the devastating news left me utterly crushed. After the ultrasound, I sat in the waiting room, waiting to see the nurse and find out what would happen next. I don't think I had ever cried like that before in my life. I felt as though all eyes were on me, and in that moment, I would have given anything for an invisibility cloak. The sorrow was overwhelming, and facing my colleagues' inquiries upon returning to work felt unbearable. To add to the turmoil, following this cancelled cycle, I developed a cyst on one ovary, annihilating any hopes of continuing the next month.

Towards the end of May 2022, my father-in-law's health deteriorated. Meanwhile, the new IVF cycle was in progress. To manage the stress, especially with the challenges in the intensive care unit at the hospital, I took sick leave and remained at home. However, this time at home only seemed to amplify my fears, particularly regarding the upcoming egg retrieval procedure. I was consumed by negative thoughts, slowly convincing myself that nothing positive awaited me. On June 18, 2022, as I sat in the waiting room before the egg retrieval, a small dose of lorazepam was working its magic. I felt somewhat intoxicated, speaking in what I thought were hushed tones, only to be told by my partner, much to his embarrassment, that I was actually speaking quite loudly and uttering some nonsensical remarks. I vividly recall the discomfort of the retrieval, despite the anesthesia and like a child, I pleaded for another dose to alleviate the pain. Thankfully, amidst it all, I felt the reassuring presence of my partner, a comforting aura that provided solace. In the end, five mature eggs were retrieved.

On June 20, 2022, we bid farewell to my father-in-law, surrounded by love and smiles. In his final moments, he assured us he'd watch over us and help us with our baby from above. Just two days later, I underwent the transfer of our only embryo. We pinned our hopes on this miracle child. This time, fully conscious in the observation room, I found solace in the serene landscapes on the walls. There was a tangible warmth in the air. In the first three days, fueled by the desire to conceive, I harbored confidence that my father-in-law's miracle was unfolding. But then, the compulsive testing began. Each day, another negative result mocked me. Cursed be that single line on the test! My intuition whispered that I wasn't pregnant, and when I confided in my partner, it sparked our first disagreement. He couldn't fathom my despair and inability to see the bright side. Days later, the nurse's call confirmed the negative blood test. The embryo hadn't even implanted. My partner remained resentful of my despair. While I mourned the loss of our potential baby, he mourned the loss of his father. I wept on the couch, he, in the bedroom, and a distance formed between us. My intuition, it seemed, had been right all along; pregnancy hadn't graced us with its presence. Damned intuition, relentless tormentor! And then there were the hormones, transforming me into a possessed cleaning fury. With my Sphynx cat hitting puberty, even a drop of pee triggered a frenzy of bleach-soaked tentacles, waging war on the foe.

In the summer of 2022, I found myself eagerly anticipating my next doctor's appointment, consumed by thoughts of the impending egg retrieval. I immersed myself in every infertility account on Facebook, scientific articles, and infertility literature. One particular piece struck a chord with me, highlighting how we are conditioned to embrace motherhood from childhood with dolls, yet fail to recognize that some of us may struggle to realize this dream as adults. During this period, our relationship was strained, and I remained oblivious to my partner's concerns. While he mourned the loss of a parent, I was tormented by my infertility, navigating through its stages of grief without fully realizing it. I found myself grappling with jealousy as I encountered countless pregnancy announcements on social media, each one serving as a painful reminder of what I yearned for. The incessant flow of baby product ads only exacerbated my distress, prompting me to contemplate severing ties with social media altogether to shield myself from these triggers. I felt suffocated by these constant reminders that another year had passed without the prospect of cuddling a little one in my arms. In an attempt to fill the void, we adopted another Sphynx cat. I suppose I satisfied my maternal instincts with these purring monsters. They brought me so much comfort that I can't help but wonder: if I spend ten years in the infertility process, will I end up with ten cats?

At the end of August 2022, I sat down with my doctor to discuss the new protocol for the upcoming IVF cycle. The prognosis wasn't promising. My doctor expressed concerns about the quality of my eggs, coupled with a low ovarian reserve. It felt like a heavy blow to my sense of womanhood. My ovaries seemed to have retired prematurely, leaving me unable to fulfill what many consider a fundamental aspect of womanhood: the ability to conceive. I grappled with feelings of inadequacy, as if I were somehow defective, yet there was no returning me to the store for a replacement. Despite the challenges posed by my poor-quality eggs and my partner's low sperm count, we made the conscious decision to forgo the option of using donors, which the doctor had suggested. The thought of carrying someone else's genetic material in my womb was something I couldn't quite reconcile with. Instead, we leaned towards the possibility of adoption should our multiple attempts at IVF prove unsuccessful.

In early September 2022, I embarked on a rigorous regimen to enhance the quality of my eggs. I decided to eliminate alcohol entirely from my life. I diligently adhered to a fitness routine, incorporating running three times a week, weightlifting, and yoga into my schedule. Furthermore, I explored the benefits of acupuncture as an additional measure. My days were filled with meticulously crafted green smoothies and thousands of supplements, all in the pursuit of optimizing my chances for success in the next IVF cycle. Immersed in a world of research and literature, I felt as though I had become somewhat of an expert in my own right.

In October 2022, I underwent the egg retrieval procedure, which yielded thirteen mature eggs. I felt a sense of pride knowing that all the efforts I had invested since September had paid off, and the doctor's newly prescribed regimen had seemingly worked its magic. Despite the significant number of eggs retrieved, I fortunately did not experience ovarian hyperstimulation. This allowed for a fresh embryo transfer, and four beautiful embryos were frozen for future use. During this period, I had taken a leave of absence from work, similar to my first IVF cycle. My partner and I had made a conscious decision to refrain from conducting any home pregnancy tests, as they tended to impact my emotional well-being. Instead, we agreed that I would wait for the blood test results, choosing to remain optimistic and trust in the process. However, I found myself succumbing to my own doubts and fears. Without my partner's knowledge, I resorted to taking multiple home pregnancy tests, all of which indicated negative results. I became consumed by this cycle of compulsive testing, so much so that I found myself purchasing more tests and conducting them discreetly at a nearby café. With each negative test, I felt as though I was spiraling further into darkness, akin to a withdrawal-stricken addict seeking solace in hiding. When I confided in a friend about my actions, unaware that she would disclose this to my partner, it only served to exacerbate the strain in our relationship. My partner's disappointment and resentment towards me became palpable, culminating in a pivotal moment where Alexandre made it clear that our relationship had reached a breaking point. It was then that I came to the blunt realization that I had lost sight of the essence of this journey—love. I had neglected my partner, failing to prioritize our relationship over the trials and tribulations of infertility. For two years, I had been so consumed by the pursuit of a successful IVF outcome that I had forgotten to find joy and contentment in the present moment. I had convinced myself that I had control over every aspect of this journey, only to be confronted with the harsh reality that I was powerless in the face of infertility. It was a painful awakening, but one that prompted me to embark on a journey of self-discovery and healing. This IVF cycle may have ended in disappointment, but it served as a poignant reminder that I needed to reclaim my sense of self and rediscover the magic within me. I had allowed myself to be consumed by despair and self-doubt, but now, I was determined to mend my shattered spirit and embrace the possibility of a brighter future.

To you, I can bare my soul... For two years, I had hidden behind these failures to the point of losing sight of myself. Unable to say what truly brought me joy, I felt like a shadow of my former self. I had to take action now to reclaim my essence, for my own sake and that of our relationship. I had long avoided the red flags raised by my boyfriend, ignored his advice. It took me two whole years to finally recognize his concerns. We had drifted so far apart that it felt as if we were strangers sharing a bed each night.

No one should ever feel that way in a relationship. Gradually, I began to embrace the art of letting go, as my partner had advised, allowing myself to enjoy the present moment. For the first time in ages, I found solace in my partner's embrace, nestled on our couch, surrounded by our beloved cats. In September 2022, amidst the ups and downs of fertility treatments, I tried to seize the moment and let go by enjoying a week-long getaway down south with my partner. Yet, despite the change of scenery, I found it impossible to shake off my anxieties about conceiving, inevitably leading to heated disagreements. In essence, my journey through infertility, combined with the pandemic, my work, our relocation to our new condo, and the loss of my father-in-law, had left numerous scars deep within me.

Consequently, I started keeping a journal of my emotions, crafting a list of negatives to purge and positives to cultivate. I've resolved to eradicate from my daily life such negative and intrusive thoughts, social withdrawal, feelings of injustice, stress, sorrow, and an obsession with motherhood, among others.

List of things to remove from my daily life:

- My negative thoughts
- Complaining
- Inner emptiness
- Social isolation
- Fatigue
- What I cannot control
- Giving up
- Blocking my emotions
- A visceral pain for not being pregnant
- Feeling of injustice
- Guilt over failures
- Life on hold during the IVF process

Things to add:

- Find meaning in my life
- Regain energy
- Rediscover my zest for life
- Only have positive thoughts
- Find new challenges
- Get out of the house
- Improve communication with my partner
- Better manage my disappointment
- Positive thoughts:
- Next time will be the right one.
- I deserve happiness.
- Wake up telling myself that today is a beautiful day.
- I am a fighter.
- I can do anything.
- I will become pregnant.

It doesn't happen with the snap of a finger. I put myself on a waiting list to see a psychologist and a mental health therapist. In the meantime, I decided to try hypnosis. I chose to broaden my horizons with a more spiritual approach. Usually, I'm more realistic and scientific. To my surprise, hypnosis helped me a lot by working on the positive aspects to add to my daily routine, by talking to myself in order to feel better. I saw a part of my dark soul and inner emptiness being trapped in a corner of the room. At the end of the session, I said "bye" to them, hoping to never encounter them within me again.

Every day, a small brick was gradually lifted off my shoulders. I felt my heart lighter. Finally! gradually, I was finding the woman I was two years ago, before this infertility process began. I can tell you that I woke up with a smile, and even after a long day of work, the smile was still there in the evening with my partner. By finding myself, I was finding my relationship. Love was coming back. In December 2022, I saw the psychologist. After my session, I had to make a list of what I love. I also suggest you make such a list. I had already started my journey which ultimately confirmed my experience of several depressive symptoms: fatigue, lack of motivation, social isolation, and absence of projects.

For two years, I hardly talked about my feelings to Alexandre. Between us, there were few conversations about our emotions. We were like aliens; we didn't speak the same language. I felt isolated in experiencing these emotions about the baby and the process itself. I tried to find support elsewhere even though expressing my feelings was never easy. When I confided in my parents, they didn't know what to say, as always. I needed their listening ear, more support, and affectionate reassurance. I wondered why those closest to me struggled to understand and comfort me. I even have a friend who hesitated to tell me that she wanted to have an abortion for fear of hurting me even more. However, connecting with a coworker and another friend who were also on infertility journeys provided some relief. Sharing our experiences and emotions through Messenger brought a sense of understanding and support I desperately needed. Coping with such a profound challenge requires a strong support system. In my case, it was limited to my partner, my closest friend, and the insights gained from therapy sessions—a fragile network for facing such adversity.

Expressing my experience through this essay has facilitated my healing. I read the lines of my thoughts to my partner, and it was at that moment that he understood what I had been feeling for the past two years. He didn't know how I had experienced those challenges. We didn't see our journey in the same way. Finally, we managed to understand each other. I suggest you talk about your feelings throughout your journey to everyone around you. Infertility still seems taboo in our society. Don't be ashamed of your situation!

Another factor that affects morale is the effect of weight gain due to hormone intake. At one point, I couldn't even look at myself in the mirror. I was far from my beautiful "six-pack" abs from before. How can I feel good in my relationship when I'm not comfortable in my own skin? By starting to feel better in my mind, I can finally, slowly, appreciate my body. We always live with several external factors that affect us, such as seasonal depression, in addition to the whirlwind of infertility.

Before, I was full of projects, always smiling, and hardly ever watched television. And then, I realized that I knew all the Netflix series, but I wasn't interested in the lives of the people around me anymore. So, every evening, I made resolutions to avoid snacking and set my alarm early for a morning workout before heading to work. Yet, these seemingly simple tasks felt like climbing a mountain. They weighed heavily on my heart, adding to the stress

I was already feeling. What used to be my daily routine now felt like an overwhelming challenge. In my early twenties, I was even training for bikini fitness competitions.

Sometimes, I find myself longing for a world of princesses and unicorns, where pregnancy happens effortlessly. I envision my period being late, deciding to take a pregnancy test, and discovering a beautiful positive sign. A moment of joy, only to be swiftly replaced by disappointment as my periods stubbornly persist on a weekly schedule, refusing to adhere to any flexibility. In the whimsical realm of fairy tales, perhaps I could forget my anguish. Unfortunately, real life doesn't afford such luxuries. And so, I must persevere in my journey of self-discovery. At times, the idea of bypassing pregnancy and embracing adoption as a solution doesn't seem so daunting. Yet, there are moments when this thought becomes all-consuming. I yearn to experience pregnancy, to feel that tiny being growing inside me, dancing in my belly. I long to experience this internal cohabitation, rather than the emptiness of a void. And one day, I hope to cradle that precious life in my arms, knowing that I would miss out on something profound if I didn't embrace this journey of unconditional love. It's a roller coaster of emotions, where both light and dark moments coexist within the span of a single day.

Slowly but surely, I began setting small goals to force myself out of the house. So, I gave myself a gentle push and went out for a drink with my best friend. It felt liberating, and I found myself smiling genuinely again. My friend was thrilled to see me in good spirits as well, and for a moment, I felt the sparkle return to my eyes. I also attempted to distract myself with a bit of shopping therapy, but the fleeting happiness it brought was short-lived. If only I possessed a magic wand to banish the lingering pain that resides near my heart and fully restore the Genevieve I once was. Even now, when I lower my head and look within, I still see a faint shadow lingering—a reminder of the void that persists within me. I long for it to be replaced by the joyous laughter shared with Alexandre, just like before. Prior to embarking on another Frozen Embryo Transfer (FET), my partner emphasized the importance of my well-being. He wanted to see the spark reignited in our relationship, reminiscent of our early days, rather than being caught in a cycle of stress and disappointment.

Gradually, I found myself smiling once more, cracking jokes, and embracing moments of joy. I still complained a lot, but it was a work in progress. In the past, I kept my emotions bottled up, maintaining a neutral facade. But with my journey, I begin to express them openly. As I pen down these words, I sense a newfound inner peace and a burgeoning feeling of well-being. It's as if spring has arrived within me, despite the winter chill outside. The inner tree of my soul is growing, and love is blossoming all around me. I now see soft pastel hues painting the world around me, and the butterflies in my stomach have returned, fluttering with excitement whenever I gaze upon my partner.

And finally, in January 2023, my appointment with the doctor confirmed my suspicions. More tests and blood work lie ahead to evaluate the chromosomes. As I ponder various scenarios, my mind races with thoughts of potential genetic issues that may prevent me from ever experiencing pregnancy.

> Should I mourn the loss of a pregnancy?
> Is my journey of infertility ending here?
> Do I need to close a significant chapter of my life?
> Is the worst ordeal of my life over?
> Do you think I should feel this way?

A few days later, I underwent a hysteroscopy and endometrial biopsy, an experience that brought some of the most intense pain I've ever felt. Unlike other medical procedures where you're typically sedated, this one required me to stay awake. Despite taking acetaminophen and ibuprofen as recommended, it felt as if I hadn't taken anything at all—the pain was relentless. With no additional pain management offered, I struggled to focus on breathing techniques as the agony consumed me. At that moment, my only wish was for my partner to be by my side, but unfortunately, he couldn't be there due to work commitments. Several days later, the discomfort in my uterus persisted, and I found myself still crying from the traumatic experience. As I awaited the results, which would take another three months to receive, I grappled with a mix of emotions—working on myself during some moments, but also battling bouts of depression as uncertainty loomed over me.

My relationship still had its ups and downs. I was so afraid that it wouldn't survive all this turmoil. Every day, it became clearer that I wanted to spend my life with Alexandre, with or without a baby. He is the one who propels me forward in life, even if I occasionally forget to enjoy life to the fullest. He reminds me of it every second. I want to laugh with him until my last breath. Alex, I will hold your hand and look you deep in your eyes: we will get through this together! I will shout it from the depths of my soul.

In March 2023, I received a call from a nurse with the results. I tested positive for anti-transglutaminases. What language is that? To put it simply, it means gluten intolerance—just another addition to my already tumultuous journey through infertility. Occasionally, I suffer from stomach pains so severe they feel like needles stabbing into my stomach, along with bloating and occasional diarrhea. I now have to wait to see a gastroenterologist for a possible diagnosis of celiac disease. Could this be the reason my little shrimp hasn't found a cozy home? Perhaps inflammation caused my body to reject the transfers. But despite this new challenge, I refuse to let it deter me. A shift to a gluten-free diet won't halt my determination.

Moreover, in the whirlwind of infertility, there always seems to be another hurdle to overcome. A few weeks later, I received another blow: chronic endometritis. A bacterium has taken up residence in my uterus instead of a baby. I'll need to endure the torment of yet another endometrial biopsy after a course of antibiotics. Bacterium, begone! You have no place here! Will the list of problems ever cease to grow? I pray with all my heart that there are no genetic issues lurking in the shadows. Help me, Almighty! Despite it all, I remain resilient. I keep smiling. We'll get through this.

When I open my medicine cabinet, my needles and syringes, sealed in their packaging, stare at me. They say to me, "When are you going to use us? We're bored. Vacation's over."

You know, I shouldn't dwell too much on my fate because life is filled with beautiful things and optimism. Almost every day on my way to work, I passed by my clinic, and each time, I couldn't wait to return there with my partner and relive that magical moment. In those instances, I felt a newfound strength running through me, empowering me to embark on another frozen embryo transfer (FET). I held onto the belief that this time, the embryo would implant and flourish as it should. I envisioned myself pregnant, enjoying the glow of happiness alongside Alexandre. We deserve it, after all we've been through. I sent out a message to the universe, a silent plea for it all to fall into place. We received what felt like a sign, a reassurance of sorts, when we heard the song "Fleur bleue" by Simon Boudreau. Additionally, with two young cats—one affectionately licking my face while the other playfully nibbles at my toes—I was no stranger to sleepless nights. So, I felt as though I was prepared for those inevitable sleepless nights with a baby.

On March 22, 2023, just before the FET, we embarked on a week-long journey down south. It was a much-needed escape, a chance to disconnect from the world and reconnect with each other. Throughout that week, it felt like we were rediscovering our love, as if we were two young souls falling in love for the first time. And then, on the beach, he got down on one knee and proposed to me. With tears of joy streaming down my face and a smile stretching from ear to ear, I said yes without hesitation. It was a moment of pure bliss, a moment I'll cherish forever. Life has a way of surprising us in the most beautiful ways. Though I may not have a diamond in my belly, I now wear one on my finger—a symbol of our love and the journey we've traveled together. I'm overjoyed to see our relationship blossoming, and every time I think back to that magical moment, I'm filled with warmth and happiness. It truly was a fairytale come true.

So, I'm still here, waiting for the stork to arrive. But as you can probably tell from my words, I'm feeling more at peace these days. I'm inching closer to that same spark we felt in the beginning. You can imagine how freeing it is to feel light and genuinely happy again. My wish for you is to experience the same. I've come to accept that some things are simply beyond our control. Right now, I'm enjoying the moment, cherishing every second with my partner. I'm sending you all my strength as you navigate your own journey. During my last egg retrieval, my embryos were starring in their own reality show. They were under constant surveillance, with cameras tracking their every move. Often, I find myself gazing at the photos of these tiny stars, imagining the day when I'll finally cradle them in my arms. It fills my heart with a radiant smile. And sometimes, I catch myself picturing my partner and our future child playing together on the living room floor, the sound of their laughter echoing through our home. For the first time in a long while, my thoughts aren't solely consumed by the idea of a baby. Instead, I'm focusing on myself and my own well-being. While I may not be able to conclude my story with news of a miracle, I want to emphasize the importance of self-care—both for your body and your mind—during the tumultuous journey of infertility. Remember to take care of yourselves, dear warriors, and keep smiling.

CHAPTER 9

ON THE WRONG SIDE OF STATISTICS

By Sarah Milette

My name is Sarah, I'm twenty-three years old, and I've been living in Montreal for three years now. I work as a special education technician in a school dedicated to individuals with intellectual disabilities or autism spectrum disorder. It's actually the reason I moved to the bustling city; I needed to gain professional experience. If someone had told me I would live in Montreal one day, I wouldn't have believed it. But I found myself embracing the big city. I can even say I've grown to love it!

Recently, I ended a relationship that had run its course. Although I'm sad, it's the sign I've been waiting for to return to my roots in Drummondville, to be close to my friends and family. There's nothing holding me back in the big city anymore. So, I bought a cozy little house, perfect for myself and my loyal companion, Paxton. All that was left was to pack my boxes and head home.

With this many changes happening, I distract myself by swiping through dating profiles. Among them, one stood out: Maxime's. I can't help but click 'Like'. Not because of his handsome smile, but because on his profile picture, he's sitting in the forest with his dog. Maxime has a beagle, just like me! Other than that, he's wearing a big hoodie, and the photo is a bit blurry.

It's nothing particularly interesting, but I can't get past his dog. With a simple compliment on his furry companion, our journey began. What started as a casual exchange soon blossomed into heartfelt conversations that stretched from dawn till dusk, and with each passing moment, I found myself drawn deeper into the enchantment of our connection.

Maxime and I finally met at the dog park. After all, it was the perfect setting for our first date! It was so cold that we each went our separate ways fifteen minutes later. After our first meeting, I wasn't particularly hooked, but he was persistent and didn't give up easily. We took several walks together. When I worked late into the evening, he offered to walk Paxton for me. I did the same with Fido when I had a day off. So, it was through our love for dogs that we found each other and grew closer. Being both passionate dog lovers, we quickly moved in together. My little house became more alive, just like our relationship and our shared projects. We repainted a few rooms in the house, built a garden in the backyard, and even adopted a third dog. What would be the next step?

I am now twenty-four years old. For several years, I relied on a hormonal IUD for contraception. This was the optimal choice since I'm quite forgetful when it comes to taking daily birth control pills. It offered a five-year solution, worry-free of unwanted pregnancy and eliminating my periods altogether. Everything was going well with the IUD until unexpected symptoms emerged. Stomach cramps and unusually tender breasts raised concerns that hadn't surfaced since I first opted for the contraceptive. Aware of the potential risk even with such a reliable method, I decided to take a pregnancy test. The result was negative. But strangely, relief was not the prevailing emotion. Instead, a sense of disappointment lingered, shared not just by me but also by Maxime, despite our short time together. In that moment, with those few words exchanged, "Let's go, let's try this," we embarked on the journey to parenthood.

I first scheduled an appointment at the local sexual health clinic to have my IUD removed. Upon arrival, I found myself laid bare, both physically and emotionally, in the care of a medical resident. Despite her efforts, the elusive strings meant for IUD removal remained beyond reach, prompting the involvement of a supervisor. As they conducted what felt like a futile "hormone fishing expedition," I grappled with a sense of discomfort and embarrassment. Leaving the clinic with a referral for an ultrasound in hand, I couldn't shake off the nagging anxiety that had settled within me. The fear of potential complications, of the IUD being lodged and causing harm to my uterus, loomed large in my mind. I remembered watching my sister navigate the challenges of fertility, grappling with polycystic ovary syndrome (PCOS) and undergoing hormonal treatments as she embarked on her journey to conceive. And so did our mother. Yet, I had convinced myself of immunity, clinging to the illusion of genetic exemption. I didn't bear a similar profile as my mother and sister. With my athletic physique and minimal body hair I believed my genetic code bestowed upon me a shield from PCOS. Also, being on contraception since the start of my periods until now, it was difficult to point out any possible anomalies with my menstrual cycle.

Thankfully, I secured my ultrasound appointment without delay and made my way to the hospital, although enduring what felt like an interminable wait in the chilly confines of a hospital corridor, clad in nothing but a flimsy gown. Despite my attempts to maintain composure, the passage of time seemed to stretch on endlessly. Following instructions to arrive with a full bladder for the ultrasound, I found myself squirming uncomfortably on the examination table, a consequence, perhaps, of adhering a bit too diligently to the directive. Eventually, the radiologist appeared, and my suspicions were confirmed—the IUD remained securely in place. I couldn't help but wonder where else it could have ventured, as its expulsion would surely have been impossible to miss. The next step in my journey led me to the gynecology clinic within the hospital, where I hoped to find specialists better equipped to address my concerns. During the appointment, a gynecology resident ventured to remove the IUD, yet encountered difficulty in doing so. Stepping in to assist, her supervisor assumed a position between my legs that left me feeling vulnerable, positioned. Despite my apprehensions, the procedure proved to be surprisingly swift and painless, in contrast with the anxiety that had plagued me beforehand. In that moment, relief washed over me like a soothing balm, grateful for the resolution of this chapter in my reproductive health journey.

Fast forward to September 2019, and I find myself liberated from the grip of hormonal contraception. Eager to reclaim control over my body and establish a regular menstrual cycle after nearly four years without any menstrual flow, I waste no time in reaching out to an acupuncturist for assistance. Witnessing the positive outcome experienced by a friend who sought similar treatment to aid in conception, fueled my determination to explore this alternative approach. I am pleasantly surprised by the results of my sessions, and quickly am able to detect my ovulation.

Despite our diligent efforts to conceive, each passing cycle brings disappointment. After two months of acupuncture treatments, we decided to allow nature to take its course. Yet, it's during this hiatus that I begin to notice troubling signs. My menstrual cycles, left to their own devices, stretch to a daunting 46 days in length. Following the advice of my sister, who navigated a similar journey years before, I turned to tracking my basal temperature in an effort to identify the ovulation peak. However, the results are inconclusive—I'm not ovulating. Faced with this obvious symptom of PCOS, I take a moment to reflect. I realize my body has been silently battling this condition for years. The gradual weight gain, the relentless cycles of acne on my cheeks—all are signs of a deeper underlying issue.

When trying to conceive a child, you're typically advised to wait at least a year before seeking medical intervention. Despite being aware of this rule, I found myself compelled to advocate for my needs sooner. I bring up the topic of my longer-than-normal menstrual cycles with my family doctor, along with my desire to start a family. Hoping for understanding and support, I instead encountered dismissal; a response along the lines of how lucky I was because many girls would like to have their periods less often. Maxime and I have to be patient. A few months later, I revisited the conversation with my family doctor, this time with a renewed determination. Though my initial reason for the visit may have been unrelated, the desire for a child remained. This time, my persistence paid off—I left the appointment armed with requests for blood work and a sperm analysis for my partner, marking a significant step forward in our journey. I wasted no time in arranging appointments for both myself and my partner to undergo the necessary tests. Additionally, learning that a referral from my doctor was not required to access the services of a gynecologist, I proactively scheduled an appointment, eager to explore all avenues available to us on our path to parenthood.

I'm twenty-five.

It pains me to realize that my dreams of motherhood remain unfulfilled, a hurtful contrast to the vision I once held for my life. A year has passed since my partner and I embarked on the journey to conceive a child. The joy of witnessing my two closest friends embrace pregnancy, their journeys unfolding in tandem, fills me with genuine happiness. Yet, beneath the surface, a small pang lingers—I would have loved to share in the joys of motherhood alongside them. Despite the setbacks, life goes on, and the hope of fulfilling our dream keeps growing. While at work, a call from Maxime shatters the fragile facade of optimism I've cultivated. Seeking the privacy of my office, I brace myself for news that will irrevocably alter our path. Maxime voice delivers the crushing blow—the results of his recent sperm analysis indicate an alteration in the parameters. A vague terminology to convey the below average number of sperm, their abnormal shape and inertia. I try my best to offer reassurance, but my tears betray the strength I want to convey. The possibility of my own infertility weighs heavy on my heart, even though I know it is beyond my control. However, empathy eclipses my own anguish as I strive to shield Maxime from the waves of guilt and despair threatening to engulf him. Together, we hold on to the hope of a medical intervention that would "fix" me, and offset the challenges posed by male infertility. As our call ends, tears cascade down my face, I'm unable to regain my composure. I knew it would be difficult for me to conceive, but the announcement of this double issue is unbearable. Anger simmers beneath the surface as I question the cosmic forces that dictate our fate: what have we done to deserve this? I summoned the courage to leave my office, masking my sorrow as best I could when bidding my colleague farewell. On the way home, grief consumes me, each sob echoing within the confines of my car. My heart aches at the thought of Maxime's pain, but I'm determined to stay strong. I must reassure him and share my unconditional love for him, regardless of the challenges ahead. For in that moment of uncertainty, one thing remains—I will never cease to love him, with or without a child.

When we get home, we're rather silent. The atmosphere is heavy with emotions. Desperately, we search for answers, but nothing comes to mind. We had never envisioned this scenario. I can't help but recall the lighthearted jokes my partner made in the days leading up to his sperm analysis; jokes about his prowess, envisioning a scenario where his efficiency might earn him the title of Quebec's very own "Starbuck" donor. How bitterly ironic it now seems. Despite this setback, we remain united and keep our focus on our dream of starting a family together.

The long-awaited appointment with the gynecologist finally arrives, and my partner stands by my side as we confront this trial together. While reviewing my blood tests, the gynecologist expresses disappointment with the lack of information she finds. To my dismay, it seems that my family doctor had only ordered a single analysis—focused solely on my thyroid gland. While the results indicate that I fall within the normal range, they tend towards hypothyroidism. The gynecologist questions the evident omission of treatment options, given the significant impact that thyroid imbalance can have on a woman's fertility.

As the appointment progresses, the gynecologist reassures me that my condition isn't cause for alarm, confident in her ability to diagnose without the need for further tests. However, she refrains from sharing her suspicions regarding my fertility struggles. The stress caused by this appointment, prevents me from asking further questions. "I'm in the presence of a professional, no need to probe any further, I can place my trust in her expertise", I thought to myself. Turning her attention to the results of my partner's sperm analysis, the gynecologist delivers a harsh reality—conceiving naturally will be a significant challenge, if not an impossibility. With a sense of urgency, she wastes no time in prescribing Letrozole, a hormone designed to stimulate ovulation in women. She explains that we'll need to undergo inseminations due to the insufficient sperm count. I'll also have to do ovulation tests at home, then call the hospital when I get a positive test to schedule an insemination two days later.

Receiving the prescription, I find myself torn between gratitude for the proactive care and the gnawing fear that this vital step might be taken too lightly. How could a treatment plan be crafted based solely on the assumption drawn from a single blood test? The uncertainty weighs heavily on my mind, prompting me to seek a second opinion from a private fertility clinic. I managed to secure an appointment with them in just two and a half months; what a relief!

In the meantime, we decide to explore an insemination procedure within the public healthcare system. Initiating hormone therapy at the beginning of my cycle, I brace myself for the roller coaster of emotions that accompanies the treatment. The onset of hot flashes, while uncomfortable, offers a glimmer of hope—a tangible sign that the medication is taking effect. However, as the days go by, impatience and agitation grip me with an intensity I hadn't anticipated. Simple mishaps, like dropping my pencil on the floor leave me on edge. At home, I cry continuously; even the presence of my partner becomes a source of irritation. I don't recognize myself.

In a moment of vulnerability, I reached out to my mother. I desperately needed a break from home, from the strain the pursuit of parenthood laid on my relationship with Maxime. I needed a night off to nurture our connection amidst this tension. This proved to be the best decision as the following days felt lighter and we rekindled.

With renewed determination, we pressed on, encouraged by the promising progress indicated by my ovulation tests and my first positive result. I immediately called the hospital to schedule my first insemination procedure. On the morning of the insemination, we found ourselves laughing as I expressed to Maxime the impression of feeling like a stuffed turkey. Despite the odd comparison, we cling to the possibility of success, the beginners' luck. In the days following the insemination, physical symptoms teased us with the promise of a positive outcome—abdominal cramps, tender breasts, and nausea all seemed to signal a possible pregnancy. Yet, the arrival of my period brought with it a crushing wave of disappointment, shattering our hopes. Between tears and heartache, we found resilience. Recognizing that success doesn't always come on the first attempt, we resolved to roll up our sleeves and try again.

We opted not to proceed with the procedures at the public hospital, as our appointment at the private clinic was scheduled shortly after. Meeting with a fertility specialist, we were met with thorough questioning about our medical histories. Upon learning of my struggles with acne and excess weight, the specialist raised the possibility of PCOS (Polycystic Ovary Syndrome). To validate these medical hypotheses and complete our dossier, a series of additional tests awaited us. For my partner, this means repeating a sperm analysis and undergoing blood tests. Meanwhile, I would undergo blood tests, an ultrasound to assess my ovarian reserve, and a hysterosonography to evaluate the condition of my uterus, tubes, and ovaries. I opted to have these tests done at the private clinic because of the lengthy waiting times in the public system. Moreover, the need for specific timing during the menstrual cycle posed a significant challenge in securing appointments at overcrowded hospitals. Embarking on this fertility journey, we embrace these initial expenses as investments in our future. I begin with the ovarian reserve ultrasound, a procedure conducted between days 3 and 5 of my menstrual cycle. Using a vaginal ultrasound probe, the doctor meticulously examines my ovaries, noting the presence of numerous follicles, raising suspicions of PCOS. Awaiting the results of my blood tests to confirm the diagnosis, I find some relief in the idea of obtaining definitive answers. With clear insights into the obstacles ahead of us, I feel strangely happy to confront the upcoming challenges, knowing nothing was left to chance or guesswork. Meanwhile, my partner is directed to consult a urologist to investigate any potential physical abnormalities contributing to the low sperm count. Following a thorough examination, no anomalies are detected. Still, he is prescribed vitamins, in an effort to improve the count and quality of his samples.

Next up was the hysterosonography, a moment I approached with a mix of anticipation and apprehension, having heard accounts of the discomfort it can entail. However, determined to maintain composure, I reminded myself of my ultimate goal in this fertility journey—to bring life into this world and experience the miracle of childbirth. I reasoned that if I could endure the pain of childbirth, surely, I could withstand this procedure.

My mother volunteered to accompany me to the clinic, alleviating any concerns about driving home afterward. As the doctor commenced the examination, I braced myself for discomfort. A catheter was gently inserted into my cervix, followed by the placement of the endovaginal ultrasound probe. With precision, the doctor injected saline solution through the catheter, facilitating a clearer view of my uterus and fallopian tubes via ultrasound. To my relief, the flux of saline solution through my tubes indicates the absence of complications. I emerged from the room with a smile on my face, as the procedure proved painless and brought positive progress in our journey towards conception.

Browsing through a support group for individuals grappling with infertility, I stumbled upon numerous accounts of successful pregnancies following hysterosonography. It seemed that the cleansing effect of the saline solution passing through the female reproductive system had proven beneficial for many women. Eager to capitalize on any potential opportunity, I waste no time in reaching out to the hospital in my area, inquiring about the possibility of scheduling an insemination for the month. To my delight, my request is met with approval, and we proceed with our second insemination at the hospital. During the procedure, the gynecologist points out the low sperm count in the sample, prompting discussions about our next steps. Despite the setback, I find solace in the reassurance that our decision to seek help from the fertility clinic was justified. The doctor remains optimistic, suggesting that the recent examination of my tubes could play a pivotal role in our favor. However, our hopes are crushed two weeks later when a new cycle begins. Despite the sadness, a part of me can't help but acknowledge a lingering sense of foreboding. Is it a defense mechanism kicking in to shield myself from further disappointment, or is it a reflection of the inadequacy of support provided by the hospital? Regardless, one thing remains clear—I resolve not to return there for insemination. Instead, we would place our trust solely in the expertise and care offered by our fertility clinic.

Once we completed all the necessary examinations, the anticipation for our meeting with the doctor soared, knowing that it marked the beginning of something truly beautiful. Finally, we will receive concrete answers and a treatment plan tailored to our unique situation. During this appointment, the doctor confirms my diagnosis of PCOS, alongside my partner's condition of moderate oligoasthenoteratozoospermia (OATS). At this point, we are informed that in vitro fertilization (IVF) stands as the most promising course of treatment, particularly given the presence of male infertility. The costs associated with this procedure are daunting: approximately ten thousand dollars for the IVF cycle, plus an additional two thousand dollars per embryo transfer attempt, not to mention the expense of medications. Though Maxime and I are prepared to invest in our dream of parenthood, we can't shake the feeling that we haven't exhausted all possibilities with insemination. Despite grappling with the loss of the romantic notion of conceiving naturally in the intimacy of our own bedroom, we want to prioritize less invasive methods that align with our desire for a semblance of normalcy. Thankfully, after a discussion with the doctor, he agrees to prescribe three cycles of insemination, after which we will need to schedule another appointment should these cycles yield no pregnancy. Leaving the meeting, we feel a profound sense of satisfaction, swiftly signing the necessary consents to proceed with the prescribed treatments.

The upcoming inseminations will be carried out under the careful monitoring of ultrasound to track the development of my follicles. Continuing with hormone intake at the start of the cycle, we'll arrange for an ultrasound before the anticipated ovulation date to assess the maturity and count of the follicles. This process, while offering hope, also increases the chance of a multiple pregnancy due to hormone-induced release of multiple eggs simultaneously. Yet, this is a risk we are willing to take without hesitation. I consider myself fortunate that my menstrual cycle aligns closely with my appointment at the clinic, allowing me to promptly notify them of day 1, filled with eager anticipation to commence the treatments. Thus begins the cycle: familiar hormonal treatments, but this time around, with meticulous monitoring of follicle development. A precise injection is then administered to trigger ovulation, ensuring the timing aligns perfectly for the insemination. Under this protocol, I underwent three inseminations, each with meticulous attention to detail. However, despite our optimism and the clinic's expertise, none resulted in pregnancy. Initially, I had believed that the detailed monitoring provided by the fertility clinic would alleviate my anxiety and instill confidence. While there is a newfound sense of assurance, the meticulous calculations also instill performance anxiety, both for me and my partner. Approaching each follicular ultrasound fills me with a constant sense of anxiety. Despite understanding that I can't influence how my body reacts to the medication, there's always the nagging fear that my follicles won't mature adequately or will remain too small. Conversely, Maxime's concerns revolve around the quantity and quality of his sperm, another aspect entirely out of our hands. Every insemination, regardless of the setting, comes with a detailed report containing the sperm count and the mobility percentage of the sample. In these times of the pandemic, Maxime isn't permitted to accompany me for the ultrasound or the procedure itself. Anxiously, he waits in the car, clutching his phone, eagerly awaiting updates on the status of his sperm sample.

A month after our latest unsuccessful insemination, we sit once again with the doctor, bracing ourselves for the familiar suggestion of IVF. However, we are encouraged to continue with inseminations using a different protocol. The new approach revolves around achieving "super ovulation" through additional subcutaneous injections, aimed at stimulating my body to produce a higher number of follicles. The target now shifts to attaining three or four follicles, but with a cautious eye towards avoiding the risk of multiple pregnancies—anything beyond four mature follicles would warrant cancellation of the insemination. Despite the inherent risks, the doctor is rather confident due to my young age. Maxime and I decide to embark on this renewed cycle of inseminations. The routine of injections becomes strangely empowering, each self-administered dose confirming we're on a whole new level. With each adjustment to the protocol, a flicker of hope reignites within me, sustaining my belief in the possibility of success. Yet, hope is a fragile thing, easily shaken. In the first insemination of this fresh series, a stark revelation affects our spirits: Maxime's sperm count is alarmingly low, a mere fraction of our previous averages. Confusion and concern grip us as even the attending doctor expresses surprise at the dismal figure. While some may opt to cancel inseminations below a certain threshold, the doctor offers reassurance: after all, it only takes one. As I lie there, post-insemination, battling back tears, my heart aches not only for our setback but also for Maxime. I know he must be even more devastated than me, while waiting in the car. We find ourselves, both saddened and confused. I know he is making a lot of effort to stay optimistic, but despite his efforts to maintain composure, I know the weight of disappointment hangs heavy upon him.

I am twenty-six years old. I'm still childless.

Yet, with each new cycle, we embrace the opportunity for another leap towards our dream. As the ultrasound probe traces the contours of my follicles, hope falters at the sight of just one. Usually, two grace my cycle. Tears spill freely as I vent my frustration to the doctor. I don't understand why I have only one follicle when medication has been added to my protocol. This is not the expected response to the quantity of hormones my body has absorbed. Recalling the bitterness of our last insemination, I'm gripped by a sense of despair. It feels like slamming into a wall. This process is so exhausting. The revelation that my lone follicle remains immature adds a layer of stress. I will have to take another day off work in two days for it to be measured again and for my ovulation to be triggered. Tears blur the distance between home and the fertility clinic, each mile a testament to the emotional toll of this ordeal. I was going to do this insemination reluctantly, my hopes dimmed by the apparent futility. I even asked the doctor if it wouldn't be more realistic to cancel the procedure and try again in the next cycle. Once again, I am told that my young age is favorable and that it only takes one. On the day of the insemination, Maxime and I are consumed by anxiety. My spirits are at their lowest due to my poor response to ovarian stimulation, and we have no idea what the sperm sample will reveal. With each attempt, Maxime must provide his sample, followed by a two-hour waiting period before the insemination. During this interval, the laboratory meticulously processes the sample, centrifuging it to enhance sperm concentration and select only the strongest contenders. In an unexpected twist, Maxime's phone rings about thirty minutes prior to the scheduled insemination. The caller from the clinic delivers a devastating blow: his morning sample yields no sperm. Despite multiple examinations, not a single trace is found. Maxime is offered to return to the clinic to produce a second sample. The news leaves us stunned, grappling with the surrealness of the situation. The weight of this revelation presses heavily upon us, straining our resolve to carry on. Watching Maxime's determined stride back to the clinic fills me with pride. His resilience astonishes me. Were our roles reversed, I might have sought solace in the sanctuary of home, succumbing to the overwhelming tide of emotions. But not Maxime. He refuses to yield, refusing to surrender to despair. Unfortunately, history repeats itself as no sperm could be found in the second sample. Following this devastating setback, we are required to consult a urologist before we can resume treatments; we need to find the reason behind our struggles. As we reflect on our journey, we come to the stark realization that what should have marked our seventh insemination is instead the seventh crushing blow we've endured. Amidst the anguish, there is a glimmer of solace: the insemination that has now been canceled was one in which I placed the least hope, wanting to cancel it myself.

The consultation with the urologist brought a wave of relief. Finally, we uncovered the reason behind the absence of sperm during our last insemination—a fever episode had been the culprit. With this diagnosis in hand, we received hopeful news: in just three months, we could resume our attempts. In reality, the waiting period had already begun, since the fever happened a few weeks ago. With summer in full swing, we enjoy the freedom to plan vacations and outings without the shadow of medical obligations looming over us. After a summer filled with beautiful adventures, we embark on what will be our last insemination. It marks the end of our journey, not because we anticipate success, but because we've reached the limits of our resources. The prospect of in vitro fertilization loomed before us, a daunting prospect both physically and emotionally. Despite my initial dread, a newfound optimism blossomed within me as we faced this pivotal step. The relentless onslaught of inseminations had taken a toll on my spirit. Never before had I felt such depths of despair. The constant battle with my body's response to medication, the toll of missed workdays, and the crushing weight of failure—all had slowly worn me down. Yet, on the cusp of IVF, a glimmer of hope emerged. This method, while drastic, holds the promise of success. We will be able to bypass male infertility, and capitalize on the advantages of my PCOS—the production of many oocytes. Hence a better chance with multiple embryos. Despite our eagerness to embark on this new chapter, we choose patience. The government's commitment to subsidize one IVF cycle per infertile couple offered a ray of hope. Maxime and I qualify for this program, and so we opt to wait, knowing that when the time comes, we'll step into this next phase with gratitude and renewed determination.

Months have passed, and despite our disappointment from previous attempts, we've come to appreciate the enforced break while waiting for Bill 73. It's given us the chance to reconnect as a couple, easing the tension that had built up. Personally, I've found solace in the cessation of hormonal treatments, giving both my body and mind a much-needed relief. Just when we've settled into this newfound tranquility, we receive the news—it's finally our turn to embark on our IVF journey. Nervously, my partner and I step into the role of chemists, carefully mixing powders into the dissolution liquid, juggling vials with trembling hands. The nightly injections become a routine, a reminder of our shared determination to see this through. My pillbox fills with medications, despite my usual aversion to taking pills. But necessity has a way of reshaping our habits. Maxime's unwavering support is my anchor through it all. He's by my side, helping me manage the medications and administering injections with gentle precision. With each passing day, I can feel the tangible effects in my belly, the fruit of our efforts being confirmed from several ultrasounds. The excitement builds as follicles multiply within my ovaries, making even the simplest tasks like fastening my pants a challenge. Despite the swelling and exhaustion that set in during the final days of ovarian stimulation, I push forward. I no longer let Maxime administer my injections; I find it too difficult. It's less painful if I do it myself, offering a semblance of control amidst the chaos. Balancing work and the demands of this process, I struggle to maintain my usual self, feeling the strain of anticipation and physical discomfort. But with each passing day, I'm reminded of the ultimate goal— to release myself from the burden of these swollen follicles and move on to the next phase of our journey.

The day of the egg retrieval has arrived. Anticipating the stress, I took a lorazepam pill the night before to ensure a restful sleep and mitigate any anxiety leading up to the procedure. Another dose is prescribed to take just before we arrive at the clinic, but taking it on the journey proves challenging. Nausea grips me as I clutch a bowl tightly, a turbulent blend of nerves and lingering hormones. Upon arrival, Maxime is ushered into a small, intimate room where he'll provide the sample, crucial for our IVF.

When he joins me in the preparation room, Maxime is dressed in a nurse's uniform while I wear the hospital gown, with nets securing our hair and blue slippers on our feet. Settled on the hospital bed, I'm guided into the operating room, Maxime is at my side. Tears blur my vision as the nurse explains the procedure and initiates vein access. Anxiety surges within me, fear of pain looming large. A cocktail of intravenous medications dulls the discomfort, leaving me in a haze as Maxime holds my hand. The doctor, holding a vaginal ultrasound probe equipped with a needle, begins the delicate task of retrieving eggs directly from my ovaries. The nurse shuttles between the procedure room and the embryologist's workstation, a flurry of activity outside my foggy awareness. Moments later, amidst the doctor's counting, I catch the first number—twenty-four eggs retrieved. Joy bubbles up within me, only to be met with the doctor's assurance that the count isn't final. The medication's effects slowly dissipate, allowing me to take in my surroundings without pain. I fixate on the television screen broadcasting images from the microscope, watching as each egg is carefully examined and processed. Still under the medication's influence, I jokingly remark to Maxime about the debris resembling olive slices. The final count arrives—thirty-four eggs—a bountiful harvest that fills us with hope for the future. Yet, back at home, fatigue and nausea weigh heavily on me. Despite my efforts to stay awake, exhaustion claims me by six o'clock. Prior to the retrieval, a nurse had explained to me that I am experiencing ovarian hyperstimulation, necessitating a two-month wait before embryo transfer to allow my body time to recuperate. Symptoms must be closely monitored, as complications could arise, manifesting as nausea, abdominal pain, fatigue, and bloating. Daily measurements of waist circumference and weight become routine, offering vital insights into my body's recovery. Any concerning changes should prompt a hospital visit.

The day following the egg retrieval, I made the decision to go to work—a choice I swiftly regretted. I felt like a human wreck, grappling with both physical discomfort and the onset of mental anguish that would persist for the next five days. Throughout the day, I relied on sips of Gatorade, as recommended by the nurses to replenish my electrolytes. My constant companion became a hot water bottle, providing a measure of relief for my abdominal pains. I await the calls from the clinic's embryologist, each one bringing a mix of hope and trepidation. On the first post-retrieval day, I received the initial update—out of the thirty-four retrieved eggs, twenty-eight proved mature and were successfully fertilized with my partner's sperm through intracytoplasmic sperm injection (ICSI). Of those, twenty-two began their journey as embryos, sparking immense joy for both Maxime and me as we dared to envision our IVF journey as a success. Comparing these results to those of other women, I imagine getting 7 embryos. However, with each subsequent call, the roller coaster of emotions intensified. On day 2, the news arrived—seventeen embryos showed promising signs of cell division, with twelve deemed of good quality. Yet, five lagged behind, casting a shadow of uncertainty over our hopes. Despite the embryologist's reassurances of about six good-quality embryos to freeze by day 5, the mounting stress weighed heavily on us and our loved ones, who shared in our anticipation of welcoming beautiful children into our lives. Then, the pivotal call arrived on day 5—four embryos had been successfully frozen, and 4 others were under observation until the next day. A sense of disappointment lingered and I'm unable to hold back my tears at the thought of the thirty-four eggs retrieved. I desperately hope to get at least one more embryo on day 6. I am already thinking ahead, and I don't know if I will have the strength to go through this process again. As I grapple with the uncertainties, the reality of our situation sinks in. The success rate of transferring one embryo is estimated at 50%, we hope to have at least two children. Yet, I remind myself to channel my energy in the present moment. My phone rings for the last time, and I am told that no embryos could be frozen on day 6. The future of our family rests on the four little embryos frozen yesterday. In the end, while our situation may not appear ideal, I remind myself that some couples must endure worse hardships. This seems to be a small consequence of the past few years of assisted reproductive technology: my mind tends to gravitate towards the negative.

I'm twenty-seven years old.

I'm closer to realizing my dream of motherhood than ever before—a prospect that fills me with excitement. My body has recovered admirably from the challenges of ovarian hyperstimulation after a week of discomfort. Today marks a significant milestone as we receive the protocol for our first embryo transfer. During this appointment, the doctor provides a retrospective of our path, shedding light on the reasons behind our modest yield of embryos compared to the bounty of eggs retrieved, likely attributed to PCOS. Despite this, the doctor shows confidence in the potential of our four precious embryos, instilling us with renewed hope. Armed with a protocol for a frozen embryo transfer (FET) on a substituted cycle, each subsequent step reignites our optimism. On day 20 of my menstrual cycle, it's time for the first step of our FET and I prepare for the first intramuscular injection—an unfamiliar territory that sets my nerves on edge. Accustomed to subcutaneous injections in the belly fold, the prospect of an intramuscular injection in the buttock muscle looms dauntingly. Fortunately, fate smiles upon me in the form of a nurse within the family—my sister-in-law—who steps forward to administer the injection. My legs feel like jelly, and I'm hot. I'm very feverish, anticipating the pain. Ultimately, everything unfolds seamlessly, and I didn't feel a thing. However, a flood of tears was unleashed. I cried for long minutes; the stress combined with the significance of this injection got the better of my emotions. At twenty-seven, I joke about being in a premature menopausal state, a side effect of the medication, plunging my body into a false menopause to facilitate the doctors' meticulous orchestration of hormonal medications, priming the terrain for the embryo's implantation. With the FET scheduled for my upcoming cycle post-injection, the next step is to wait for my period. As the days pass by, I find myself anxiously awaiting the arrival of my period. Alarmed by its absence, I reach out to my fertility clinic, hoping for some reassurance. Though a pregnancy test yields a negative result, I cling to the hope that this delay is merely a hiccup, devoid of deeper implications. I'm consequently requested at the clinic for an ultrasound. In a sobering moment, the screen reveals the unwelcome presence of two cysts, nestled on one of my ovaries—uninvited guests disrupting the delicate balance of our journey. Too sizable to ignore yet not menacing enough to evoke immediate concern. I'll have to return to the clinic in about ten days to monitor the progress of these unwanted guests. The weight of this news settles heavily upon me. Just as I dared to envision the finish line of our marathon, fate throws another hurdle in our way. It's a stark reminder that the path to parenthood is seldom linear. I cling to the fragile hope that these cysts will dissipate on their own because the doctor mentioned the possibility of prescribing birth control pills for a few months to offer my ovaries a rest. A paradoxical strategy in the pursuit of conception!

In the interim, I keep an appointment for acupuncture—an initiative originally intended to nurture my uterus in preparation for the FET. Despite the unwelcome presence of cysts, I choose to proceed, recognizing the opportunity to establish a trustful connection with my acupuncturist. To my surprise, this seasoned practitioner offers reassurance, suggesting that acupuncture can aid in the absorption of the intruding cysts while also alleviating the stress that often accompanies medical procedures. As she strategically places needles at various points on my body, I find myself enveloped in a sense of calm upon leaving the session. My next ultrasound appointment was moved up since my period arrived in the meantime. I anxiously await my turn in the clinic's waiting room. The scan reveals that while the cysts persist, they've significantly diminished, no longer posing a barrier to the impending embryo transfer. The long-awaited green light fills me with joy; my FET will take place this month. I find it hard to believe that we might finally see the light at the end of the tunnel. With meticulous care, I organize my pillbox, determined to navigate the medication regimen with precision. Concurrently, I continue my acupuncture sessions, finding solace in the sense of empowerment this ritual offers, instead of just enduring the various effects of the medication. As I start the series of progesterone injections, Maxime assumes the role of caretaker, administering the injections with tenderness. His dedication speaks volumes, a tangible manifestation of our shared commitment to this journey. In his involvement, he feels that he can make a difference, he finds purpose.

On September 8, 2022, Maxime and I embarked on a poignant journey to the clinic, to bring back the precious cargo of our embryo nestled within the depths of my belly. It's a swirling mix of beautiful emotions. Before setting out, we pause at a baby store, a symbolic pilgrimage in preparation for our impending parenthood. Together, we select a delicate muslin cloth—a small yet significant token, symbolizing the tender nurturing of our little one. Our choice settles on a charming blanket adorned with a mushroom house motif—soft, warm, and delightfully gender-neutral.

As I cradle this tiny blanket close to my heart, we make our way, light hearted, to the fertility clinic. In the procedure room, it's time to meet our embryo. While personal effects are typically prohibited in this sterile environment, the compassionate nurse makes an exception, allowing me to keep our cherished blanket close by. As the last patients of the day, the risk of contamination is minimal, offering a rare moment of comfort amidst the clinical setting. On the screen before us, they first show me an identification label, asking me to confirm my identity. Once this formality is done, the embryo is unveiled—a perfect 3AA grade, poised for its journey towards implantation, its delicate shell already beginning to crack open in a gentle hatching. The medical team marvels at its beauty, its perfection—a testament to the wonders of life unfolding before our eyes. A whimsical coincidence emerges as the nurse remarks on its resemblance to a mushroom, mirroring the motif on our chosen muslin cloth—a subtle yet profound connection that fills us with hope and gratitude. At this moment, I dare to believe in the signs that destiny might be weaving our path towards parenthood—it's our baby, our miracle, coming home.

Following the transfer, I'm granted a ten-day sick leave—a precautionary measure due to the risks posed by my job to a potential pregnancy and because, medically, a woman is considered pregnant post-transfer until proven otherwise. Returning home with our precious bundle of joy, we feel lighthearted; a long-awaited feeling. I carry the blanket with me everywhere, a tangible symbol of our future, a beacon of light illuminating the path towards our long-awaited miracle.

The next morning, I wake to a sobering reality—a fleeting moment of happiness swiftly replaced by the weight of doubt and apprehension. Despite my good intentions to foster positivity, a lingering voice of skepticism persists, questioning why this time would be any different. It's a familiar dance of hope and despair—a defense mechanism born from years of disappointment and dashed dreams. Despite my best intentions, I struggle to envision the fairy-tale ending I so desperately long for. Five days post-embryo transfer, I find myself seeking distraction in a TV series. I squirm on the couch, struggling to find a comfortable position when my body betrays me with the familiar twinge of menstrual cramps and a dull ache in my lower back. There's a sinking certainty in my gut—my period is imminent, and with it, the crushing realization that the little embryo has chosen another path. With tears in my eyes, I reach for a pregnancy test. Negative. With trembling hands, I place the test abruptly on the counter, knowing that I might want to see it again later. I've often rummaged through the trash to reanalyze a pregnancy test. This time, I refuse to be deceived. Climbing the stairs to bed, I send a solemn message to my partner telling him that we won't be calling him "dad" just yet. Exhaustion weighs heavily upon me as I drift into a fitful sleep, tears silently staining my cheeks. As I go down to the living room, my swollen eyes betray the silent anguish of earlier hours. I retrieved the pregnancy test. To my bewilderment, a faint second line now graces the test. With trembling hands and a heart heavy with emotion, I call Maxime. The only words I manage to utter are "I don't understand." In a desperate bid for clarity, I send him a photo of the test, clinging to the fragile hope that I'm not hallucinating. Not used to analyzing such faint pregnancy tests, it takes him a while to tell me that he sees two lines. Since Maxime works with my brother-in-law, I can hear him seeking counsel from this experienced parent. I grapple with a torrent of emotions, clinging to the faint glimmer of hope offered by that elusive second line. I hastily make my way to the pharmacy. Armed with five boxes of early detection tests from a trusted brand, I return home with a singular determination—to unravel the mystery behind that faint line once and for all. As soon as I get home, I conduct the test, each passing second stretching into an eternity as I await the verdict. And then, in a moment suspended in time, a beautiful pink line emerges. I keep repeating the same phrase, like a broken record: "I don't understand."

Unable to contain my joy, I eagerly shared the photo of the pregnancy test with my mother, sister, and, of course, my best friend. That faint line, barely discernible yet bursting with promise, heralds the realization of a cherished dream. It carries joy, excitement, and the possibility of dreaming again about future projects. In the quiet moments of anticipation, I can already imagine my rounded belly in photos in front of the Christmas tree, the gentle kicks of the baby distorting the curve of my belly, and our miracle nestled snugly in a baby carrier during our outdoor adventures. It's a symphony of hope and anticipation, a canvas painted with the hues of newfound joy. Each morning brings with it a ritual of anticipation as I eagerly await the results of yet another pregnancy test and share them with my family; equally eager to hear the daily update. I love watching the test soak up. With each pink line that blooms within the window of the plastic stick, I find myself bathed in a sense of perpetual satisfaction. Ten days post-embryo transfer, I make my way to the hospital for the pivotal blood test that will confirm my pregnancy. Despite the lingering feverish anticipation, I wait anxiously for the nurse's call. And then, in a moment that fills me with unbridled joy, I'm met with the words I've longed to hear—my blood test is positive, I am pregnant. However, my hCG level is not particularly high. I am at 63 when a pregnancy in a gray area is situated at 50 or less. They try to reassure me; the important thing is simply that my level has doubled in 48 hours. Once again plunged into the depths of intense stress, I anxiously count the days until the next blood test. The phone call finally arrives, delivering the long-awaited news that my hCG levels have risen to 158. I can finally breathe. I whisper a silent plea to my unborn child—hold on, my baby, hold on tight. The next milestone is a viability ultrasound at the seventh week of pregnancy—a moment of truth that will reveal whether our hopes are indeed anchored by the presence of a tiny, beating heart. The weeks that follow the blood test have been filled with emotions: swirling currents of joy, tempered by jets of fear. The scars of our fertility journey run deep, leaving me haunted by the specter of past disappointments and always expecting the worst. At work, I am reassigned to more administrative tasks. I appreciate the calmness that these new functions provide me.

Today, at 7.3 weeks pregnant, Maxime and I hit the road for Montreal—a day etched with both anticipation and trepidation as we prepare to lay eyes on our little miracle. The weight of uncertainty hangs heavy upon me, each passing moment fraught with the delicate fragility of this newfound joy. My name echoes in the waiting room. It's our turn. I am escorted to the ultrasound room. Stripped of my pants and underwear, I can't help but hope this is the last time. The doctor begins the ultrasound and examines my ovaries before moving to my uterus. With each passing second, the tension mounts, amplified by the gravity of the doctor's solemn expression. I have no idea what I'm supposed to see on the screen, but I can sense the news isn't good. Summoning the courage to voice my fears, I tentatively inquire, "There's no heartbeat?" A heavy silence descends as the doctor conducts his examination. Finally, I hear his words, like a crushing blow to the fragile string of hope that still cling to my heart: "It's over", he murmurs, his voice laced with sympathy. The fetus inside me stopped developing towards the end of the fifth week of pregnancy. The doctor will prescribe medication to help me evacuate my miracle. My partner holds my hand, as stunned as I am by the devastating revelation. Alone in the examination room, we grapple with the enormity of our loss, words failing us in the face of such profound grief. I put my clothes on, I can't even cry. We sit in silent mourning, enveloped by the weight of our sorrow, unable to talk, we await the nurse who will guide us through the painful process of inducing a miscarriage. The minutes seem endless. A few tears finally trickle down my cheeks, but I hold them back because we are sitting in a crowded room. When the nurse finally appears, her gentle demeanor offers a semblance of comfort. Yet, even her empathetic words fail to ease the relentless ache that gnaws at my soul. I wonder when I will wake up from this nightmare. Given a prescription for Misoprostol, I am confronted with the harsh reality of what lies ahead—a painful and agonizing journey to bid farewell to the little embryo that once held our hopes and dreams. I can't help but wonder, perhaps this tiny miracle sensed the love that awaited it, choosing to linger a little while longer in the warmth of my embrace.

On the journey home, we remain silent, both trying to assimilate the news and begin our mourning process. Ironically, the radio seems to echo our sorrow, only playing a sad soundtrack. It's as if the universe itself mourns with us, offering its condolences in the form of melancholic melodies. In addition to my grief, I find myself grappling with an additional burden—the weight of expectation. Our families, who supported us throughout this journey, eagerly anticipate our news. The date and time of our ultrasound appointment were marked on everyone's calendars. Summoning the last vestiges of strength that reside within me, I steel myself to deliver the heartbreaking news:

Hello!

I just want to let you know that our journey ends here for now. Our embryo stopped developing at 5.6 weeks. I don't feel like talking right now, so I'm going to turn off my phone. I'll get back to you when we've managed to understand what's going on! Xx

Later in the afternoon, at my request, the fertility clinic reaches out with the results of this morning's blood test. My HCG level, a mere 2975, falls short of the expected range for this stage of pregnancy. It's a bitter pill to swallow, yet somehow, it leads me slowly towards the path of acceptance. Despite the crushing weight of reality bearing down upon me, I can't bring myself to take the prescribed Misoprostol. A stubborn glimmer of hope flickers within me, clinging desperately to the belief that perhaps, against all odds, the pregnancy might still be viable. The thought of relinquishing what little remains of this precious hope fills me with an inexplicable sense of dread. As I brace myself for the physical and emotional onslaught that lies ahead, I go ahead and follow the prescribed regimen—painkillers to numb the pain, followed by the insertion of the Misoprostol tablets. I should expect to have cramps and bleeding within the next twelve hours. If not, I will have to take a second dose of Misoprostol. Yet, despite my best efforts, the medication yields no discernible effect, leaving me trapped in a limbo of uncertainty and anguish. The following morning, I made an appointment for urgent care with my family doctor to request a sick leave. How could I face going to work with an impending miscarriage, not to mention the psychological distress. I can't fathom the thought of providing support at work. Gratefully, my family doctor grants me a month-long respite from the burdens of daily life. What a real relief! I know this sick leave will help me, even though emotionally, I feel like I'm in denial.

I feel neutral, empty. I don't know if I should curl up and cry in my bed, but I can't resolve myself to do it. Thankfully, my family doctor has agreed to follow up with me regarding the miscarriage. This will save me the trouble of traveling to Montreal in such a sensitive context.

Upon returning home, I brace myself for the second dose of Misoprostol. Hours tick by, yet there's no change. It's disheartening to realize that even medication fails to initiate the inevitable miscarriage, despite knowing it won't lead to the birth of a child. My numerous conversations with the fertility clinic yield little solace, as they urge patience, citing the unpredictable nature of Misoprostol. This only heightens my anxiety, leaving me feeling utterly helpless as I grapple with the uncertainty of the situation. Every twinge and sensation in my body becomes a source of relentless scrutiny, as I desperately try to decipher any sign of progress. Though I've begun to experience some bleeding, it's not substantial enough to expel the embryo. It's probably due to stopping the progesterone injections. Amidst a flurry of appointments at both the fertility clinic and with my family doctor, an ultrasound confirms that the sac still remains attached. Despite my repeated pleas for a dilation and curettage (D&C), I'm met with bureaucratic hurdles, each moment prolonging the agony of carrying a lifeless embryo within me. When the fertility clinic finally agrees to my request for a D&C, they provide me with a list of specialized women's health centers, primarily equipped for voluntary pregnancy terminations. It's a stark reminder of the gravity of my situation—having to consider such drastic measures for a child that was once so fervently desired. In the end, I turned to my gynecologist, presenting her with my request for a D&C. After fasting for the remainder of the day, I wait anxiously by the phone, bracing for the call that will usher me into the hospital. Thankfully, the wait proves not to be in vain, as

I'm granted the much-needed relief of a same-day D&C. As I prepare to undergo the procedure under general anesthesia, a sense of reassurance washes over me. Despite the gravity of the situation, I find solace in the prospect of drifting into a painless slumber, knowing that when I awaken, this devastating chapter will finally be behind me. The medical staff's exceptional care and compassion provide a glimmer of comfort amidst the turmoil, as they extend a rare gesture of allowing my partner to accompany me into the preparation room.

Post-surgery, I began to feel a sense of relief, both mentally and physically. The operating room marked a significant turning point, bringing an end to the uncertainty that had plagued me. Slowly, I emerged from my self-imposed isolation, opening myself up to the warmth of family and friends once again. Life resumed its course, and we found ourselves ready to embark on the journey of fertility treatments once more. Thankfully, my pregnancy hormone levels swiftly returned to baseline, meeting the necessary criterion for a second embryo transfer. Following this, I revisited my fertility doctor, who recommended an endometrial biopsy to ensure there was no inflammation. Given the potential risk of endometritis following the D&C, it was a cautious measure to mitigate any further complications. The biopsy results coincided with the onset of my menstrual cycle, revealing a healthy endometrium. With this reassurance, I was deemed ready for my second Frozen Embryo Transfer (FET). Despite my excitement, a sense of apprehension lingered within me. I approached this FET with a newfound detachment, perhaps as a defense mechanism against potential disappointment. Gone were the wooden marks for cycle photos and the symbolic blankets. My optimism was tempered by the sobering reality of past experiences and the estimated 50% chance of implantation. Scheduled for Friday the 13th, a day often associated with misfortune, my transfer stirred a mix of emotions. Yet, in the days following the procedure, a bit of optimism emerged. However, it was short-lived as I experienced small electric shocks in my cervix and menstrual cramps, a familiar sensation from the first pregnancy. On day 9, post-ovulation, Maxime and I nervously took a pregnancy test, bracing ourselves for the outcome. Though initially hesitant to look, we eventually examined the test together, spotting the faint second line. Surprisingly, it was my partner who noticed the second faint line first, and then I saw it as well. Yet, instead of jubilation, the sight of the positive test reignited painful memories of my previous miscarriage, casting a shadow over the prospect of a new pregnancy.

Filled with anxiety and apprehension, I continue to take daily pregnancy tests, like the first time. First promising sign, the blood test confirms rising hormone levels. What if this time was the one? A second blood test confirms that the pregnancy is progressing. I'm Irritable and on edge until the viability ultrasound, overwhelmed at the uncertainty of what lay ahead. I scrutinized every symptom, or rather the lack thereof, convincing myself that this pregnancy was just a product of my imagination. As we made our way to the fertility clinic, irritability consumed me, and even my partner's presence felt like an intrusion on my inner turmoil. I yearned to fast forward time, wishing I could teleport, to skip past the uncertainty. Upon arrival at the clinic, we are directed into an ultrasound room. I undressed and settled onto the examination table, cocooned in a flimsy paper drape. Maxime's restless pacing only added to my agitation, and I snapped at him sharply, desperate for a moment of calm. A knock on the door startled me, and my heart raced as the doctor entered the room, introducing himself:

— "Hello, I'm Dr. X. I will be performing your ultrasound today. How are you feeling?

— Terrified.
— Oh, I see. Is it because of what happened last time?
— Yes, it was very difficult.
— Well, let's take a look right away. Please, lay down."

The doctor inserted the ultrasound probe and positioned himself between the TV screen and me, preventing me from seeing the screen. Then, he quickly announced:

"Everything looks good. Take a look!"

As the doctor steps aside, he reveals the most incredible sight: my baby, my miracle, on the ultrasound screen. Seeing that tiny heartbeat flickering fills me with overwhelming emotion, and tears stream down my cheeks uncontrollably. It's a moment of pure disbelief and joy—despite bracing myself for the worst, here I am, receiving the most beautiful news imaginable. The doctor meticulously takes measurements of our little miracle, and with each reassuring detail, my belief solidifies. I am truly, undeniably pregnant! My partner squeezes my hand tightly, his eyes shining with emotion. In that moment, amidst the tears and overwhelming happiness, I couldn't imagine feeling any more complete. Leaving the clinic this time, it's with a profound sense of accomplishment and victory. Suddenly, this place holds a different, brighter significance for me. And as we share the news with our families, I know that this time, our announcement will bring nothing but joy and celebration. The cloud of sadness that once hung over us has finally lifted.

Upon arriving home, I wasted no time in reaching out to my gynecologist to secure my first prenatal appointment. The days stretch ahead, seemingly endless, until the two-week mark when I'll have my first follow-up. Despite witnessing the miraculous sight of my baby's heartbeat, a lingering fear gnaws at me, whispering of potential collapse. I search desperately for signs of pregnancy, grasping at any subtle changes. A faint tenderness in my breasts and the slightest shift in bedtime routine become my only indicators. Throughout the day, I find myself instinctively pressing against my chest, seeking reassurance that my little one is still thriving within me. Ironically, I catch myself yearning for the discomforts of nausea, wishing for tangible proof of this new life growing inside me. Yet, there are fleeting moments of clarity when I remind myself to cherish each passing day. But my miscarriage has left its mark, stealing away the innocence of joyous anticipation. Perhaps one day, I'll reclaim the joy of pregnancy fully. But for now, I navigate this delicate journey with a heart weighed down by the echoes of the past.

For my initial prenatal appointment, Maxime accompanies me, a comforting presence amidst my nerves and jitteriness. Anticipating a small dating ultrasound from my gynecologist, I hope it will ease my apprehensions. After initial discussions with the nurse, I'm ushered into the examination room to meet the gynecologist. As she flips through her notes, she recalls our previous encounter during the D&C procedure. I share my anxieties about being here again and embarking on another pregnancy journey. To calm me down, she suggests I lie back for an ultrasound, my first abdominal one. A wave of relief washes over me as we witness a strong heartbeat and measurements indicative of a healthy progression. After the ultrasound, we reconvene at her desk, delving into more detailed discussions about pregnancy while also scheduling routine first-trimester blood tests. I make a request for prenatal screening blood work, eager to uncover the gender of our miracle baby. Little did I know at that moment, I was so naive to think that everything could be fine.

A week later, I headed to my appointment for the prenatal screening blood work. The clinic outlined the timeline for receiving the results: an email if all appeared well, a call from my gynecologist if there were concerns about Down syndrome. In the days that followed, I found myself compulsively refreshing my inbox, each minute feeling like an eternity. Then, a private number lit up my phone screen. My heart sank as I answered, fearing the worst. It was indeed my gynecologist on the line, prompting an immediate rush of worry. "Oh no, does my child have Down syndrome?" She confirmed having received our results and urged me to meet her at the hospital for further discussion. I dialed Maxime, my voice trembling as I shared the news. Despite her attempts at reassurance, we both braced ourselves for difficult revelations. Maxime, fortunately, worked close to home, and we converged at the hospital, our anxiety palpable in the waiting room. Surrounded by other expectant mothers, I couldn't help but feel a stark contrast to their joyful anticipation. Irrationally, I found myself apologizing, as if bearing responsibility for our unforeseen challenges. Our turn came and we entered her office. After a brief exchange, the gynecologist broached the subject directly. The blood test revealed a heightened risk of Down syndrome. Yet, there was a glimmer of hope in the statistical analysis: based on my age and my partner's age, the test held a 56% likelihood of accuracy. We clung to that remaining 44%, clinging to the possibility of a favorable outcome. The next day's nuchal translucency appointment loomed, offering a chance for further insight. The doctor, conducting a swift ultrasound, noted a concerning thickness in the baby's neck. Despite her efforts, capturing a clear image proved challenging amidst the baby's incessant movements. Finally, with a heavy heart, she confirmed our worst fears: an increased nuchal translucency measurement, dimming our hopes for a positive prognosis. The gynecologist's demeanor mirrored our somber mood, her optimism noticeably diminished. This pregnancy was so eagerly anticipated. I had envisioned joyous moments like a gender reveal, surrounded by loved ones. But reality intruded, and we opted to learn the gender immediately. Thus, I carry within me a precious little girl, likely with Down syndrome. It is the very announcement that was sent in a message to our families. I won't have the opportunity to do a gender reveal; it will be more of a diagnosis reveal.

We received a referral to a specialized neonatology hospital for further genetic testing and care for high-risk pregnancies. Within days, we secured an appointment, but in the interim, my partner and I found ourselves grappling with profound and challenging discussions, confronting our differences of opinion head-on. It was crucial for us to navigate this journey together, respecting each other's opinion while seeking a common path forward. We needed time to absorb the news, to reflect, and ultimately, to come to a decision that would bring us both peace. Ultimately, we resolved to continue the pregnancy, embracing the notion of welcoming a child with special needs into our lives. However, we also established a boundary. If our baby were to show additional signs of developmental abnormalities that would compromise her quality of life, we would not prolong the pregnancy. It was a decision made with careful consideration and deep concern for both her well-being and ours. With this resolve, we attended our genetic counseling and high-risk pregnancy follow-up. From the outset, we expressed our position, and we were met with understanding and compassion. Following discussions with a genetic nurse, we proceeded to the ultrasound room. There, a radiologist meticulously examined our little girl, followed by a doctor who provided further insights. The news was sobering. Our daughter's nuchal translucency was indeed elevated, corroborating the results of the blood test for Down syndrome. Additionally, a cystic hygroma, a swelling of fluid around the baby's head and neck, was discovered. We were informed of the varying outcomes this condition could entail, from self-resolution to potentially fatal consequences. We were sent home with plans for a follow-up at sixteen weeks to perform an amniocentesis. What started as hope and determination now gave way to profound disillusionment. Anxiety and disappointment cloaked us in silence as we made our way home. When we finally found the strength to speak, it was to acknowledge a painful truth: we had reached the threshold we set for our baby's physical development. The wait until the next appointment loomed like an insurmountable hurdle, one my mental health could not bear. What torture to think that the life I carry could be snuffed out at any moment, without me even me knowing it's happening.

Upon returning home, I reached out to the high-risk pregnancy nurse to convey our decision: we were opting for a medical termination of pregnancy (MTP). Eventually, the doctor returned my call. Sensibly, we agreed to take the weekend to deliberate, avoiding hasty decisions amidst the emotional tumult. She promised to reconnect on Monday. Over the weekend, emotions were running high. I felt like I had lost the determination that my partner had. A part of me felt it was over, I was unable to relish the pregnancy anymore, unable to appreciate the first images of my growing belly. Yet, another part clung to hope. Despite the odds, our child remained steadfastly attached. When the doctor called on Monday, she suggested meeting later in the week, understanding my fragility and the uncertainty of reaching sixteen weeks. For Maxime and I, it was a good compromise to mutually respect our differences of opinion. Quite surprisingly, the next morning brought an urgent call, summoning me to the hospital without delay. Despite being short of the required weeks, they accommodated me for an amniocentesis. In any case, if we opted for an MTP, the risks associated with the hasty procedure would have no impact. With Maxime away, my mother stepped in to accompany me. Though a different doctor greeted me, the procedure mirrored the previous one—a thorough ultrasound followed by a consultation. This time, the conversation brimmed with reassurance, infusing me with the hope to persevere. According to the doctor, the hygroma is likely to resolve itself as it is not large and is still well connected to the baby's neck. I was presented with 2 options for diagnosing Down syndrome. I could either undergo a chorionic villus sampling biopsy immediately or wait the sixteen weeks mark and have an amniocentesis performed. After discussing with Maxime over the phone to assess the risks, we opted for a chorionic villus sampling biopsy, seizing the chance despite the higher risk of miscarriage. The subsequent forty-eight hours were a nightmare. Enduring cramps and stress, I weathered the crucial period post-procedure, relieved to emerge unscathed. As my phone rang, the genetic nurse delivered the initial biopsy results, confirming Down syndrome. While not unexpected, the news brought solace, confirming the absence of any rare genetic issue and marking a step forward in our journey.

Finally, encouraged by the doctor's hopeful outlook on the cystic hygroma, Maxime and I found the strength to continue the pregnancy. Though cautiously optimistic, we harbored a slight reservation until the viability ultrasound, mindful of the unpredictable nature of our daughter's development. Nevertheless, we've wholeheartedly embraced her uniqueness, resolved to dedicate ourselves to ensuring she enjoys the best possible quality of life. Now, when I catch a glimpse of my burgeoning belly in the mirror, I can't help but smile. I dare to believe that the worst is behind us.

More than our longing to cradle you in our arms, we recognize your own tenacity, your will to persevere and thrive.

We are one in six couples experiencing infertility.

We had a one in five chance of experiencing a miscarriage. Although it happened, you decided to stay.

We had a one in 1208 chance of having a child with Down syndrome according to my age.

We had a high risk of Down syndrome in the blood test, but a 56% chance that it was a true positive.

We had a 0.35% chance of you having a cystic hygroma.

And yet, here we are!

I may not have luck with lotteries, but I've certainly hit the jackpot when it comes to defying the odds. This wasn't exactly what your father and I envisioned when we first learned of your tiny presence nestled in my belly, but here we are, poised to embrace an atypical journey as an atypical family. Eugénie, believe me when I say that you are not just awaited, but deeply cherished and longed for. After years of grappling with infertility, you have chosen us as your family, and in return, we choose you, wholeheartedly and without reservation. Maxime and I are ready to open our hearts and arms wide for you, just as our families and loved ones eagerly await your arrival. Eugénie, we can't wait to explore the world with you, to witness every discovery and share in every joy. From the depths of our souls, we already love you, each precious chromosome, from the crown of your head to the tips of your toes.

CONCLUSION

"I'm sorry I'm late to the baby shower..." A simple text message I sent to a friend, while going through my own challenges. Not only was I missing an important event in my friend's life, but I was also losing myself in the dream of my own baby shower, beaming with a radiant smile and a beautifully round belly...

The journey through fertility treatments is a peculiar kind of magic, placing you in the front row of life's creation. From acupuncture, meditation, and an arsenal of vitamins to witnessing the embryo entering your uterus on a screen—this moment is surreal. The path is fraught with highs and lows, much like the mountains we sometimes encounter in life. Initially, it was hard to accept the small joys my partner and I would miss: the thrill of a spontaneous positive pregnancy test, the joy of surprising our family, or the excitement of that first ultrasound. The first ultrasound (which I hope to experience one day!) must be both terrifying and exhilarating, especially in the context of IVF, where positive thoughts are vital to combat the underlying anxiety.

Acceptance and grief are inherent to my journey, but so are love, passion, and happiness. I've realized that this arduous path is not just my story but a way to help other women on similar journeys. Writing this book, creating a community, and assisting eight other women in sharing their stories has been a blessing. This is why I faced infertility—to help others. Without IVF, this book wouldn't exist, this community wouldn't be formed, and crucial conversations would remain unspoken. My journey indeed has a greater purpose.

One particular day stands out vividly in my memory. I was sitting in a café, furiously scribbling in my journal, trying to capture the emotional whirlwind that had become my constant companion, while waiting for my friends. I was meeting Alex and Annabel for a quick coffee chat. That moment revealed the profound power of vulnerability and the strength that emerges from sharing our stories. I found myself opening up about the painful journey I was on and listening to Annabel's story. Now a mother of three, her strength gave me hope. Both Alex and Annabel infused me with the energy needed to share my story and create this magical book.

One year later, Annabel was moving to Europe with her family, Alex was traveling with hers, and I deeply missed our coffee dates. Secretly, I harbored a dream of surprising them in Europe during the summer, proudly sporting a big round belly. It remains a cherished dream...

From the inception of this book to today, seven out of the nine women featured have become pregnant and are expecting their babies soon! Andrée-Anne and I are still navigating this journey, but we continue to hold on to hope.

Strength and resilience are the core themes of this book. The ability to rise from adversity, to face the storm with courage and hope, is what defines each woman's journey through infertility. These stories are not just about enduring pain but about finding joy and purpose amidst the struggle. They are about the laughter that follows tears, the friendships born from shared pain, and the unyielding hope that propels us forward.

To every woman who has read this book and found solace, thank you. Your strength, resilience, and hope drive this project. Remember, you are not alone. We stand together, stronger and more hopeful for the future.

It is imperative that we continue to talk about our fertility, our health as women, and make it a priority in today's society. For our friends, our families, and our future daughters, we must ensure these conversations happen openly and frequently. By doing so, we can create a world where no woman feels isolated or shamed for her journey, but rather empowered and supported. This is our mission, and together, we can make a difference.

GLOSSARY

Infertility: The inability to conceive a child despite regular sexual intercourse for a period of one year or more.

Sterility: Total inability to conceive a child.

IVF (In Vitro Fertilization): Assisted reproductive technique where eggs are fertilized in a laboratory.

ICSI (Intracytoplasmic Sperm Injection): Assisted reproductive technique where a sperm is injected directly into the egg.

FET (Frozen Embryo Transfer): Assisted reproductive technique where frozen embryos are transferred into the uterus.

Endometriosis: A condition where tissue lining the inside of the uterus (endometrium) grows outside the uterus.

PCOS (Polycystic Ovary Syndrome): A condition where the ovaries produce excessive amounts of male hormones.

Egg donation: Process by which eggs from a donor are used for fertilization.

Sperm donation: Process by which sperm from a donor is used for fertilization.

MFI (Male Factor Infertility): A condition where a man's immune system attacks his own sperm.

Blastocyst: A developing embryo that has reached a specific stage of development before implantation.

Transvaginal ultrasound: Imaging procedure that uses sound waves to produce images of the inside of the vagina and pelvic organs.

Embryo: A fertilized egg that develops into a human being during the early weeks of pregnancy.

Endometrium: The lining of the inside of the uterus responsible for embryo implantation.

Fibroids: Non-cancerous tumors that develop in the uterus and may interfere with pregnancy.

Follicles: Fluid-filled sacs in the ovaries where eggs mature.

Ovarian hyperstimulation syndrome: An excessive ovarian response to hormonal stimulation that may occur during fertility treatments and can lead to medical complications.

www.ingramcontent.com/pod-product-compliance
Ingram Content Group UK Ltd.
Pitfield, Milton Keynes, MK11 3LW, UK
UKHW020656030925
7703UKWH00043B/1089

9 782982 014039